THE DASH DIET COOKBOOK FOR BEGINNERS:

The Complete Guide To Prevent And Avoid Hypertension, Without Giving Up Appetizing And Healthy Dishes

With 200 Easy & Tasty Heart-Friendly Recipes And A 28-Day Meal Plan

D1606886

Tara Cohen

Table of Contents

Introduction

Are you one of the many people unknowingly living with high blood pressure? You're not alone. About one in three adults suffer from this condition. The good news is that a diagnosis of high blood pressure doesn't mean that you're destined for a life of prescription medication. It's relatively easy to lower your blood pressure naturally, especially by improving your diet.

Whether you've been diagnosed with high blood pressure or you're just hoping to prevent it from developing in the future, a diet for high blood pressure is one of the most important things to address. A healthy diet is the key natural remedy for high blood pressure, especially since it is completely safe, simple, and works quickly to improve your overall health in addition to your blood pressure.

Although not a real disease, high blood pressure (hypertension) is among the main risk factors for cardiovascular disease, one of the leading causes of death in the world.

It is a widespread condition in industrialized countries. In the United States alone, about 7 million people die each year from various diseases that are primarily caused by hypertension. Men and women are equally likely to develop this condition during their lifetime.

Men are more likely when they are younger, before turning 45, than women. The probability reverses after age 65 when women's risk becomes higher than men's. Hypertension is an easily treatable condition, but it can cause serious health damage if ignored, increasing the chances of heart failure, heart attacks, and strokes.

What is High Blood Pressure

Blood pressure is the force of blood pushing against the walls of the arteries as it is pumped by the heart. High blood pressure occurs when this force is greater than normal. There are often no obvious symptoms of high blood pressure, even when readings reach dangerously high levels. Because of this, many people don't know they have it.

However, when blood pressure rises, some warning signs may include:

➢ Chest pain
➢ Mental confusion
➢ Headaches

- ➢ Irregular heartbeat
- ➢ Ringing in the ears
- ➢ Vision changes (black vision or bright dots in front of the eyes)
- ➢ Nosebleeds (nosebleeds)

When you experience symptoms, you are likely experiencing a hypertensive crisis, which is considered a medical emergency that requires immediate treatment.

Hypertension is dangerous because it makes the heart work harder than necessary, and the increased blood pressure against the walls of blood vessels can damage arteries and organs, such as the heart, kidneys, brain, and eyes.

In many cases, hypertension has no symptoms, so much so that it is called the silent killer; if not recognized and managed, it can cause:

- • Kidney disorders
- • Blindness
- • Heart attack.

How Can Prevention Be Done

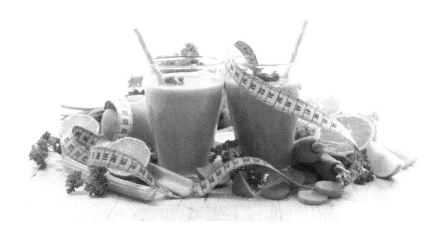

Some people who has high blood pressure, may not have experienced any symptoms. It's essential to remember that you can control your progress and improvement through diet and lifestyle changes. Taking steps to improve your health can make a significant effort to slow or prevent blood pressure disorders and enhance your quality of life.

Focus on Weight Loss

Losing weight is one of the most common reasons for going on a diet. Carrying excess weight contributes to high toxicity levels in the body by storing toxins instead of releasing them through the kidneys.

There are some necessary and easy changes you can make to shed those first pounds, which will begin to help you onto the path of regular weight loss:

- Drink plenty of water. If you can't drink 8 glasses a day, try adding unsweetened natural sparkling water or herbal teas to increase your water intake.

- Lower the amount of sugar and carbohydrates you consume. It doesn't require adapting to a ketogenic or low-carb diet – you'll notice a significant change after ditching soda and reducing the bread and pasta by half.

- Take your time to eat and avoid rushing. If you need to eat in a hurry, grab a piece of fruit or a small portion of macadamia nuts. Don't eat sugary and salty foods as much as possible. Choose fresh fruits over potato chips and chocolate bars.

- Create a shortlist of health-friendly foods, that you enjoy and use this as your reference or guide when grocery shopping. It will help you stock up on snacks, ingredients, and foods for your kitchen that work well within your DASH diet plan, at the same time reducing your chances of succumbing to the temptation of eating a bag of salted pretzels or chocolate.

Once you make take a few steps towards changing the way you eat, it will get easier. Making small changes at first is the key to success and progress with a new eating and living way.

Quit Smoking and Reduce Alcohol

It's not easy to quit smoking or using recreational drugs, especially where there has been long-term use and the effects have already impacted your health. At some point, you'll begin to notice a difference in the way you feel and how your body changes over time. It includes chronic coughing related to respiratory conditions, shortness of breath, and a lack of energy. These alterations may be subtle at first, and it may appear as though there is minimal damage or none at all. However, smoking inevitably catches up with age and contributes to cancer, premature aging, and organism damage. The more toxins we consume or add to our body, the more challenging it becomes for the organism to work efficiently, which eventually slows their ability to function.

Reducing smoking on your own, or switching to e-cigarettes or a patch or medication, can help significantly over time. Setting goals of reduction until the point of quitting can be a beneficial way to visualize success and provide a sense of motivation. The following tips may also be useful for quitting smoking and other habit-forming substances:

Join a support group and talk to other people who relate to you. Share your struggles, ideas, and thoughts, which will help others and yourself during this process.

Track your advancement on a calendar or in a notebook, either by pen and paper or on an application. It can serve as a motivator, as well as a means to display how you've done so far and where you can improve. For example, you may have reduced your smoking from ten to seven cigarettes per day, then increased to nine. It may indicate a slight change that can be kept in mind to focus on reducing your intake further, from nine cigarettes to seven or six per day, and so on.

Be aware of stressors in your life that cause you to smoke or use substances. If these factors are avoidable, make every effort to minimize or stop them from impacting your life. It may include specific people, places, or situations that can "trigger" a craving or make you feel more likely to use it than usual. If there are situations that you cannot avoid, such as family, work, or school-related situations, consult with a trusted friend or someone you can confide in who can be present with you during these instances.

Don't be afraid to ask for help. Many people cannot quit on their own without at least some assistance from others. Seeking a counselor or medical professional's guidance and expertise to better yourself can be one of the vital and essential decisions you make to improve the quality of your life.

Getting Active

The fundamental ways to keep fit and healthy is by staying active and engaging in regular exercise. Regular movement is key, and exercise is different for everyone, depending on their abilities and options. Fortunately, there are unlimited ways to customize an exercise routine or plan that can suit any lifestyle, perhaps low impact to start, or if you're ready, engage in a more vigorous workout. For many people experiencing high blood pressure, one of the significant struggles is losing weight and living a sedentary life. The movement is generally minimal, and exercise is usually not commonly practiced. Smoking, eating processed foods, and not getting the required nutrition can further impair the body, so that exercise is seen as a hurdle and a challenge that is best avoided. Making lifestyle changes is not something that should be done all at once, but over some time – especially during the early stages – so that the condition's impact is minimized over time and becomes more manageable.

Where can you begin if you haven't exercised at all or for a long time? For starters, don't sign up for a marathon or engage in any strenuous activities unless it is safe to do so. Start slow and take your time. Before taking on any new exercise or activity, always talk to your doctor to rule out any impact this may have on other existing conditions, such as respiratory conditions, as well as heart health.

Most, if not all, physicians will likely recommend exercise as part of the treatment plan but may advise beginning slowly if your body isn't used to exercise.

Simple techniques to introduce exercise into your life require a commitment. It can begin with a quick 15-minute walk or jog and a 10-or 15-minute stretch in the morning before starting your day.

Best Advice to prevent

As specified, you can prevent blood pressure diseases through diet, but other general lifestyle factors will help. As a rule, you need to follow a lifestyle that keeps your body weight under control and makes you feel healthy. Here are some tips:

> **Exercise Regularly**

As we said above, it is essential to be physically active to keep your heart and breathing system healthy. Most doctors recommend exercising 2-3 times a week and performing mild exercises to keep yourself active but not too tired or exhausted. Three hours in total of mild exercise per week is excellent for this purpose.

> **Monitor Your Blood Sugar Levels**

Blood sugar levels and diabetes are often a side effect or even a contributing factor to blood pressure problems. Even if you don't currently have diabetes, it is still essential to monitor your blood sugar levels to further place you at risk of developing diseases. Check them at least once a month and if you are in pre-diabetes or full set diabetes status, make sure that you take all the medicines that your doctor prescribes for your case.

> **Keep Your Immune System Balanced**

When our immune systems are underactive or overactive, many types of diseases can occur due to the body's inability to fight them properly. In the case of high blood pressure, some autoimmune conditions like Lupus are negatively associated with the disease's progression. In this case, your doctor may prescribe steroids to keep your immune system from getting over-triggered and attacking blood and vital organs.

How To Improve Your Diet To Lower High Blood Pressure

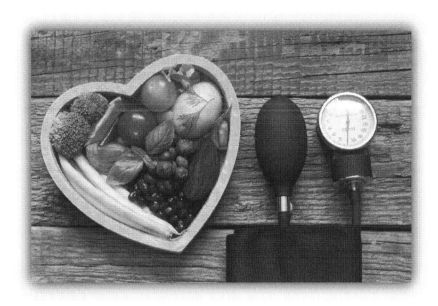

Research shows that about 50 percent of people with high blood pressure fail to control their condition, either because they aren't aware of the problem or haven't made lifestyle changes that promote overall heart health.

It may seem daunting to overhaul your entire life to help control your high blood pressure - for example, taking prescriptions, eating differently, reducing stress, and exercising. But you'll be happy to know that it's usually surprisingly easy for many people to help deal with high blood pressure just by making a few simple changes.

For example, people who follow a high blood pressure diet like the DASH diet over time have been able to lower their systolic blood pressure by seven to twelve points, a significant amount that can make a big difference. This can be accomplished in steps through very simple actions, such as eating more fresh produce and cooking more often. You can help fight high blood pressure by taking these steps:

- Recover your fitness weight
- Doing moderate physical activity almost every day

- Follow a healthy diet, including foods low in sodium, and rich in potassium
- Do not overdo alcoholic beverages

Eating a nutrient-rich, minimally processed diet can help bring your blood pressure closer to normal or even within a perfectly healthy range. You will start to see a difference within a few months, but consistency and continuous effort, is the key.

Foods, including fresh vegetables and fruit, lean proteins, and some healthy fats, help reduce inflammation and prevent nutrient deficiencies, which are two of the main causes of high blood pressure. And a healthy diet for high blood pressure is even more effective when other lifestyle changes are made, such as managing stress better, exercising regularly, quitting smoking, and getting a good night's sleep.

Obviously, it is very important to point out that if you have hypertension and need to take medication, you should strictly follow your doctor's orders.

The importance of reducing salt

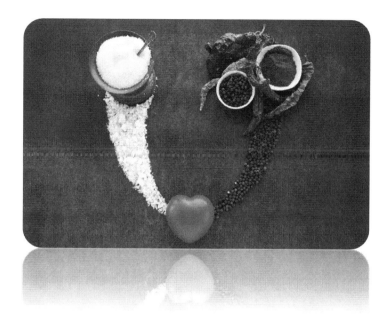

When we talk about diet and hypertension, the accent inevitably falls on cooking salt and on foods that contain it in significant quantities. We know that the incidence of the disease is lower in populations that adopt a low-sodium diet. Therefore, a diet rich in sodium increases the risk, therefore the probability, of developing hypertension, but it is not said that those who blatantly break this rule will suffer from hypertension, and those who respect it will be exempt.

The role of sodium is in fact blurred by many other predisposing factors, such as dietary habits in the broadest sense (excess calories and lipids favor the appearance of the disease), genetic predisposition, sedentariness, and lifestyle (stress, smoking, alcohol or drug abuse, etc.).

Both in the preventive and therapeutic field, the diet for hypertension is based on four fundamental points

- containing the intake of sodium (low-sodium foods)

- increase potassium intake (through a generous consumption of fruits, vegetables, and whole foods)
- control body weight and limit alcohol consumption.

Sodium intake should be reduced below 3-5 grams per day, thanks to the reduction of salt consumption (or its replacement with low-sodium similars) and foods rich in sodium. In this regard it should be remembered that one gram of normal cooking salt contains 400 mg of sodium; therefore, a pinch of salt contains about one gram of sodium, whereas a teaspoonful contains 5 grams, a spoonful 15, and a fistful 30.

How to Reduce Salt Consumption

Limiting the addition of salt to foods may seem difficult, but actually, there is nothing simpler; the palate can be educated, and if the reduction is done gradually, it will get used to the new diet without too many problems, finding tasty dishes that until recently seemed bland; salt can also be replaced with low-sodium products (containing, for example, potassium chloride) or various aromas and spices, such as hot peppers, herbs, garlic, parsley, rosemary, sage and oregano. In this sense, parents have a great responsibility towards their children, who should be directed, since the very first years of life, to a diet low in snacks and appetizers rich in salt.

Once the addition of sodium has been reduced, it is also necessary to reduce the consumption of foods in which it is present in large quantities; packaged food and cured meats, for example, are two of the main obstacles to reducing sodium in the diet. Moreover, these are generally high-calorie foods, which increase the stimulus of thirst, often quenched with sugary drinks or alcohol. Beware also of stock cubes and preparations to flavor dishes - very used in restaurants, especially in oriental ones - because they are rich in monosodium glutamate.

Some of the best foods that lower blood pressure naturally

Vegetables

Eating a variety of vegetables is a staple for every diet that exists, considering that vegetables are high anti-oxidation foods full of protective nutrients like fiber, vitamin C, vitamin K and various electrolytes (but very low in calories). Leafy greens like spinach, kale, mustard greens and turnip greens are potassium-rich foods and among the healthiest foods on earth, and they add almost no calories to your diet.

Fresh Fruit

Consuming fresh fruit (as opposed to juices or sugary canned fruit) is a great way to increase your intake of fiber, electrolytes like potassium and magnesium, and antioxidants like flavonoids and resveratrol, especially fruits like berries, citrus, kiwi, apples, and cantaloupe.

Lean proteins

This can include foods such as seafood caught in the wild and meat from free-range, grass-fed animals. This type of protein is important for maintaining your energy levels up and for satisfying your diet. It makes you feel full, balance your blood sugar and helps maintain muscle strength.

Beans and legumes

Beans and legumes are great sources to increase your intake of fiber, protein, B vitamins, and some antioxidants. They're suitable for those who don't consume meat or animal products, have low calories, and are almost completely sodium-free (if you make them from scratch or rinse the canned ones well).

A helpful tip to make beans even healthier and more digestible is to soak them overnight before cooking, in water and lemon or apple vinegar , which helps release anti-nutrients that block mineral absorption and interfere with digestive processes. In this way, you can consume beans/legumes several times a week as an appreciable alternative to meat.

Healthy Fats

Nuts and seeds are a potent source of healthy fats, and they also add protein and fiber to your diet. Aside from seeds and nuts, other beneficial anti-inflammatory foods that are full of healthy fats include avocados, coconut oil, and extra virgin olive oil. These fats help stabilize blood sugar levels, a benefit that helps keep you full and less likely to overeat.

Whole grains

The DASH diet recommends whole grains, mainly because they are a good source of fiber and certain minerals known to lower blood pressure, especially compared to refined carbohydrates.

Organic and unsweetened dairy products

The DASH diet includes low-fat or fat-free dairy products such as milk and yogurt. It is important to focus on the quality of the dairy products you consume. Choosing organic, unsweetened, ideally raw dairy products, and from Grass-Fed footed animals is the best choice for your overall health, even more so if you suffer from hypertension.

The Dash Diet

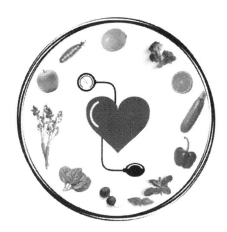

If you have blood pressure dysfunction, a proper diet is necessary for controlling the amount of toxic waste in the bloodstream. When toxic waste piles up in the system and increased fluid, chronic inflammation occurs, and we have a much higher possibility of developing cardiovascular, bone, metabolic, or other health issues.

What Is A Dash Diet Is All About?

A Dash diet is designed to reduce the level of toxic waste in the body. It also means controlling and adequately minimizing the number of toxins that go into your body with each meal. It is done by eliminating the intake of the main culprit behind the abnormal increase of toxic waste in our blood – sodium.

The improper eating habits of most people out there, particularly those in the western part of the world, are why we always see a high increase of sodium levels in the body, which is the main reason behind the rise of blood pressure problems. Salt intake is a primary culprit behind toxic waste in the body, but also processed and preserved foods, hide an incredible amount of sodium that is even more harmful than salt itself.

How This Diet Works?

The DASH diet is mainly aimed at improving health by keeping blood pressure at bay: it is useful both in prevention and in case of existing problems with hypertension. Potassium, calcium, fiber, and protein are considered the key nutrients for keeping blood pressure at the right levels, but it is also important to keep the sodium content of foods on this diet low.

A typical Dash diet consists of lots of fruit, vegetables, pulses, cereals, and nuts. Many people who follow this diet also add chicken and low-fat dairy products. This diet leads to many benefits:

- Prevents excess fluid and waste buildup

- Prevents the accumulation of waste and toxins in the bloodstream

- Decreases the likelihood of developing other chronic health problems, e.g., heart disorders

- It has a mild antioxidant function in the body, which keeps inflammation and inflammatory responses under control.

- It helps build and maintain healthy bones.

- It can also treat many diseases and is safe for most people to use.

- Losing weight is another good reason to follow a Dash diet.

The benefits mentioned above are noticeable once the patient follows the diet for at least a month and then continuing it for more extended periods to avoid relapses.

Why It Does Well?

The Dash diet is good because it will help build a strong foundation for one's health. It is a well-known fact that heart failure is one of the leading causes of death every year. Proper intake of nourishing foods that contain essential vitamins, minerals, and nutrients and cleaning your body from harmful infections is a right and promising way to prevent such chronic conditions.

How Can It Positively Affect For You?

Some nutrients play a significant role in a Dash diet , why they can influence your state of health. Essentially, the Dash diet is based on balanced consumption of certain nutrients like potassium and sodium, and the right amount of macronutrients.

Potassium

Potassium is a mineral that naturally occurs in certain foods and plays a role in regulating heart rhythm and muscle movement. It is also needed for keeping fluid and electrolyte balance at normal levels.

Sodium

Sodium is a trace mineral found in most foods that we eat today, and it is the key component of salt, a sodium compound mixed with chloride. Most food that we consume and specially processed food is positively loaded with salt; however, we may be eating sodium in other forms, e.g., fish.

The key role of sodium is to regulate blood pressure, regulate nerve function, and maintain the balance of acids in the blood. However, when sodium is excessively high, and the body can't expel it, it can lead to symptoms like an elevated feeling of thirst, swelling of hands, feet, and the face, high blood pressure, and problems with breathing. It is why it is suggested to keep sodium intake low to avoid the above.

Protein

Protein is a nutritional compound that consists of amino acids, which play a key role in various system functions like cell communication, oxygen supply, and cellular metabolism. They are also a part of a healthy immune system.

Protein itself is not an issue for us. The fact is that, when protein is metabolized, waste by-products are also created and are filtered through the kidneys. This waste, after will be expelled through urine.

When kidneys cannot filter out excess protein, it gets accumulated in the blood and causes problems. It doesn't mean that one should avoid protein totally, as it is necessary for some metabolic functions, as long as it's taken in moderate amounts and choose proteins of high biological value.

Carbohydrates

Carbohydrates act as a key source of fuel for our bodies. The consumption of carbs is turned into glucose in our system, a primary energy source.

Carbs are okay to be eaten in moderation in case of high blood pressure and normally the daily recommended allowance is up to 150 grams/day. However, persons whit these problems, should control their carb consumption to avoid any sudden spikes in their blood glucose.

Fats

Our bodies' fats act as energy sources, release hormones, and regulate blood pressure in balanced amounts. They also carry some fat-soluble vitamins such as A, D, E, and K, which are also very important for our systems. Not all fats are equal though some are good for our health, and some are bad. Bad fats are saturated and trans fats found in processed meat, dairy, processed foods, and other products. They are also found in margarine and vegetable fat shortening. It is highly recommended to limit eating food with saturated and trans fats to avoid any cardiovascular problems, e.g., elevated blood pressure and clogging of the arteries. It's better to opt for Omega 3 fatty acids, which are found in caught fish and are also well supplied by walnuts, hazelnuts, almonds, and seeds, e.g. flax, sunflower, and sesame.

Losing weight with the DASH diet. What to do in practice

The DASH diet, in combination with other lifestyle changes, can help you prevent or control high blood pressure. If your blood pressure is not too high, you may be able to keep it under control simply by:

> ➤ changing your eating habits
> ➤ losing weight if you are overweight
> ➤ exercising regularly
> ➤ reducing alcohol consumption.

The DASH diet has other benefits too, such as reducing LDL cholesterol (the so-called 'bad' cholesterol), another cardiovascular risk factor. Recent research has shown that it is possible to lose weight if you follow the DASH diet and reduce your sodium intake.

If you are trying to lose weight, try to achieve a lower calorie threshold than you usually consume. Don't forget to follow these tips to save more calories:

- Use non-fat or low-fat condiments, so industrial butter should be eliminated and replaced with ghee or clarified butter. Extra virgin olive oil is usually the ideal choice.

- Halve the amounts of seed oil, margarine, mayonnaise, or sauces, or, if they exist, choose low-fat versions.

- Gradually get used to smaller portions.

- Choose skimmed or semi-skimmed milk or milk products.

- Check labels to compare the amount of fat in packaged foods: foods claiming to be low-fat or fat-free can sometimes have a higher calorie content than normal foods due to their sugar content.

- Moderate quantities of very sweet foods, such as cakes, processed yoghurt, sweets, ice cream, pudding, fizzy drinks, and fruit juices.

- When eating (low-fat) yoghurt, add some fruit.

- As a snack, choose fruit, some chopped and cleaned vegetables, unsalted and not too greasy popcorn, or rice cakes.

- Drink water or tonic water, flavoured with a twist of lemon or lime.

- Combining the DASH diet with a regular exercise programme, such as running or swimming, will help you to lose weight and maintain results in the long term; half an hour a day of moderate-intensity exercise can be a real panacea.

If your blood pressure is a little higher than average, walking at a brisk pace almost every day for half an hour may be enough to keep you off medication.

Even if you do not suffer from hypertension, physical activity can still help keep you healthy. If your blood pressure is in the normal range but you are sedentary, the likelihood of suffering from hypertension increases, especially with age, overweight, obesity or diabetes.

To start with, the physical activity programme can simply consist of a walk around the block for 15 minutes, once in the morning and once in the evening. In order not to lose motivation, gradually build up your programme and set yourself new goals. Remember that trying to do everything at once can cause health problems and thus force you to stop.

If you suffer from chronic health problems, or if there is a history of heart disease in your family at a young age, I recommend that you seek medical advice before starting any exercise programme.

The 5 Steps to Eat Good

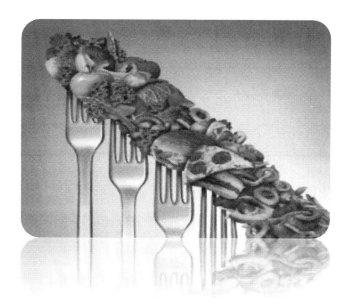

The below steps will allow you to eat directly as you deal with your recovery path.

Step 1: Choose and Plan Nourishments with Less Sodium and Salt

Look for nourishments for which the label reads: sodium underneath 300mgs for every serving, and the ingredient list has sugar (under the title sugars) less than 25 grams or less than 5 grams of saturated fat. Take note: buy the greater part of your nourishment uncooked. Try to purchase whole grains, unfilled pasta, and new products likewise. Stay away from the canned and prepackaged nourishments. Here are a few tips:

- Purchase new and fresh food frequently. Sodium (a piece of salt) is added to many arranged or packaged foods you purchase at the general store or cafés.

- Cook foods without any preparation instead of eating arranged foods, "fast" food sources, frozen meals, and canned food sources that are high in sodium. At the point when you set up your very own foods, you control what goes into it.

- Use flavors, herbs, and sodium-free instead of salt.

- Check for sodium on the Nutrition Facts name of food bundles. A Daily Value of 20% or more means the nourishment is high in sodium.

- Try lower-sodium adaptations of solidified meals and other comfort foods.

- Wash canned vegetables, beans, meats, and fish with water before eating.

- Search for food names with words like sodium-free or salt-free, low, decreased, no salt or sodium, or unsalted or lightly salted.

Step 2: Eat the Perfect Amount and The Correct Types of Protein.

Many diet experts recommend trying to get your protein from natural products like chicken, fish, white meat, eggs, and lean red meat. It is incredibly essential to ensure that you are getting the correct protein measure at every meal. Try to achieve 16- 20grams of protein each meal session. Which doesn't mean 20 grams of meat or fish or eggs (consider that roughly 100 grams of any protein food contains within it about 20 grams of protein). Consider that about 100 grams of any protein food contain about 20 grams of protein, so it can mean 250/300 grams of meat, fish, eggs, per day. If you have a low protein intake, obtaining protein from protein powders can supplement a deficiency.

Step 3: Choose Food Healthy for Your Heart Health.

Maintain a heart specialist's authorization before beginning any change in your old dietary intake. You ought to also keep in mind that solid fat or processed sugar can raise cholesterol levels. What unites blood pressure disturbances, heart disease and kidney disease is pollution with chlorine in the drinking water; therefore, when it comes to drinking water, consider low-mineral or lightly mineralized water with a fixed residue of between 50 and 500 mg/l, alternating with water low in sodium. In choosing healthy food for your heart, stay away from everything that provides extra sodium and fluid and, i.e., sodas, processed and junk foods, along with bacon, sausage, cheeses, cakes, pies, white bread, white rice, and fish.

Step 4: Choose Foods & Drinks with Less Phosphorus

An excessive concentration of phosphorus in the blood is not to be underestimated, as it can lead to the formation of small mineral deposits in organs and tissues. The parts affected by calcifications could be the heart, skin, lungs, joints, and blood vessels, leading to diseases, like hypertension and cardiovascular problems. You should also be particularly careful with products that are not very fresh: from meat to preserved cheeses, soft drinks, and frozen foods, as they have phosphorus salts added to enhance the flavor of the food and to preserve it better.

Step 5: Choose Foods with The Right Amount of Potassium

Why? It supports nerves and muscles to function properly. Potassium is a key mineral for restoring healthy blood pressure balance in the body, and when you don't have enough potassium, symptoms of high blood pressure can start to emerge. Conversely, increasing the amount of potassium-rich foods in the diet can lead to a reduction in high blood pressure.

Getting started!

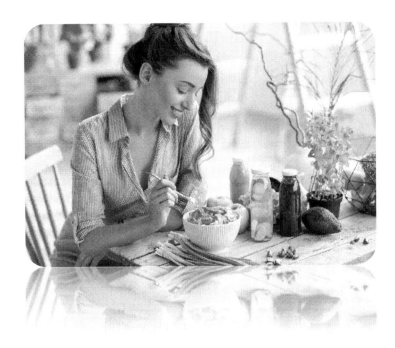

Getting started on the DASH diet is very simple. Here are some tips to help you:

Change your habits gradually.

- If you now eat only one or two portions of vegetables a day, add one portion at lunch and another at dinner.

- If you are not used to eating fruit or if you only drink fruit juice at breakfast, add a portion at meals or eat fruit between meals, trying to eat whole fruit, rich in fiber.

- Gradually replace whole milk intake with skimmed or semi-skimmed milk and try to make sure you consume dairy products or cheese up to three servings per day, always from grass-fed animals. If you have problems digesting milk and milk products, try taking tablets containing the enzyme lactase (available in pharmacies); alternatively, buy lactose-free milk. Alternatively, buy a vegetable milk, such as rice, coconut, almond.

- If you can, make your own sauces and salad dressings at home. In any case, read the labels of dressings and sauces to choose those with the lowest sodium content, and avoid trans and saturated fats.

- Consider meat as part of the meal, not as the heart of the meal, and vegetable side dishes as the heart of the meal.

- Limit your meat intake to around 200 g per day - there is no need to eat more. Eat about 100 g at each meal, which is about the weight of a pack of cards.

- If you are used to eating large portions of meat, gradually reduce them by half or by eating about a third of what you are used to.

- Have at least two vegetarian meals a week.

- Increase the portions of vegetables and legumes in each meal. Replace white pasta and white rice with whole wheat pasta and brown rice.

- Favor fresh fruit or other foods low in saturated fat, trans fat, cholesterol, sodium, sugar, and calories as desserts or snacks outside of meals.

- Fruit and other low-fat foods offer a wide variety of flavors. Use fruit preserved in its own juice or water, rather than fruit in syrup. Fresh fruit is easy to eat. Dried fruit is handy to have in your bag or car, ready for a snack.

- Try a different snack: unsalted rice biscuits, nuts, and sultanas, whole meal crackers, low-fat yogurt, raw vegetables.

- If you're not used to drinking water, start making herbal teas, and consume 3 or 4 cups a day. Gradually it will start to become a habit. And then you can alternate it with large glasses of water, never cold, never from the fridge, preferably warmed, maybe with lemon juice in it.

- Keep a record of everything you eat and your physical activity habits before starting the DASH diet to take stock after a few weeks.

What Nutrients Are Needed and Needed to Avoid

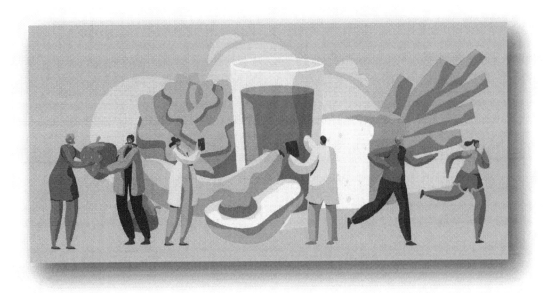

Many foods work well within this diet. Once you see the available variety, it will not seem as restrictive or difficult to follow. The key is to focus on foods with a high level of nutrients, making it easier for the body to process waste by not adding too much that it needs to discard. Balance is a significant factor in maintaining and improving a long-term health.

Daily nutritional goals

The following nutritional goals are for a food plan of 2100 calories per day:

- ➢ Total fat: 27% of calories.
- ➢ Saturated fat: 6% of calories.
- ➢ Protein: 18% of calories.
- ➢ Carbohydrates: 55% of calories.
- ➢ Cholesterol: 150mg.
- ➢ Sodium: 2300mg*.
- ➢ Potassium: 4700mg.

*1,500mg of sodium was tested as a minimum target. It was found that if lower, it's even better for lowering blood pressure. This was found to be especially effective for middle-aged and elderly people, African Americans, and those who had previously suffered from hypertension.

Nutrients That Are Needed

The DASH plan shown below assumes a daily intake of 1800 calories. The number of servings in each food group may vary from person to person from those listed, depending on calorie requirements. This can be a cue to use when planning your subsequent menus.

➢ **Cereals:**
- Daily servings: 2.
- Broken down into meals= 1 slice of bread, 30 g dry cereal, 1/2 cup cooked rice, pasta, or cooked whole-grain cereal.
- Important to know about the DASH diet: these are the main sources of energy and fiber.
- *Examples*: whole wheat pasta, brown rice, red rice, black rice, bulgur, quinoa, amaranth, oats, rye, rice galette, whole wheat bread, cereal bread.

➢ **Vegetables:**
- Daily servings: 3-4.
- Break down into meals: 250 g of raw leafy green vegetables, 250 g of sliced raw or cooked vegetables, 1/2 cup of vegetable juice.
- *Examples:* Starchy vegetables - These are potatoes that have been soaked to reduce the starch content if needed. Mixed vegetables also include corn and peas, but you'll need to eat them less often because they have a high phosphorus content. Non-starchy vegetables - Onions, beets, carrots, spinach, Swiss chard, arugula, valerian, turnips, turnip greens, celery, broccoli, asparagus, green beans, red and green peppers, summer squash, eggplant, iceberg lettuce, kale, raw spinach, radishes, cabbage, cucumbers, leeks, turnips, cauliflower, Brussels sprouts, mustard greens, red and green peppers, broccoli.
- Important to know about the DASH diet: they are rich sources of potassium, magnesium, and fiber.

➤ **Fruit:**

- Daily servings: 2-3.
- Break down outside of meals: 1 medium fruit; 1/4 cup dried fruit; 1/2 cup fresh fruit; 1/2 cup fruit juice.
- *Examples:* apples, apricots, bananas, dates, grapes, oranges, grapefruit, mangoes, cantaloupes, pineapples, grapes, strawberries, kiwis, tangerines, oranges, pomegranates, blackberries, blueberries, raspberries, pears, plums, watermelon, cherries, kumquats, kiwis, oranges, tangerines. Again, apple juice, apple mousse, grape juice, and low-sugar blueberry juice, centrifuges.
- Important to know about the DASH diet: a rich source of potassium, magnesium, and fiber.

➤ **Skim or fat-free milk and dairy products:**

- Daily servings: 1- 2.
- Servings: 1 cup milk or yogurt, 45 g cheese.
- *Examples:* skim or part-skim milk; low-fat, or low-fat cheeses (quark, cottage cheese); low-fat yogurt.
- Important to know about the DASH diet: these are important sources of calcium and protein.

➤ **High-protein foods:**

- Meats, cheeses, and eggs - These are eggs, lean cuts of meat, poultry (from grass-fed animals), fish and seafood, cottage cheese which should be limited due to high sodium content, low cholesterol egg substitutes.
- Important to know about the DASH diet: these are important sources of minerals, amino acids, and protein.

➤ **Beverages:**

- These are homemade teas and herbal teas, water (also flavored with lemon, mint, and cucumber, or fruit), vegetable broths.
- Important to know about the DASH diet: these are essential for hydration and important sources of vitamins and minerals.

Food Items to Be Avoided

We have already listed everything that is harmful and most of it is salty and sweet, industrially produced foods. The list includes sweetened and carbonated drinks, industrial fruit juices, beer, water sweetened with fruit juices, syrups, baked goods, candy, condiments, ice cream, honey, molasses, salted nuts, regular chocolate with sugar, canned meat, canned foods, normal table salt (which we will replace with whole-grain sea salt or Himalayan pink salt), frozen pizzas, ready-made sauces, ready-made marinades, salty chips and salty snacks, salami, bacon, industrial cheese, pepperoni, corned beef, sausage, hot dogs, bacon, lard, industrial butter, sweetened whipped cream, margarine.

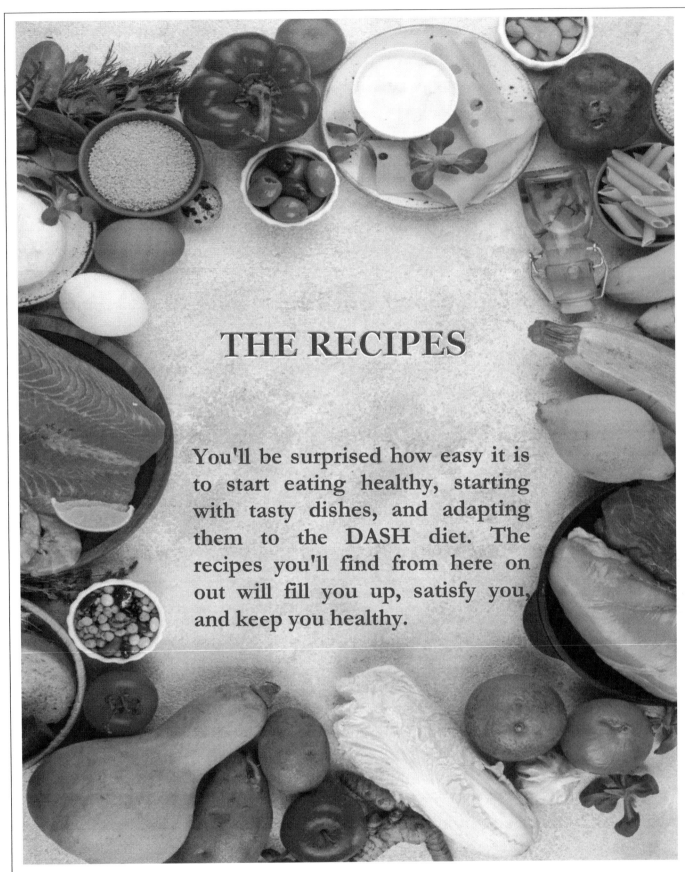

THE RECIPES

You'll be surprised how easy it is to start eating healthy, starting with tasty dishes, and adapting them to the DASH diet. The recipes you'll find from here on out will fill you up, satisfy you, and keep you healthy.

Healthy and tasty versions of sweet and savory breakfasts

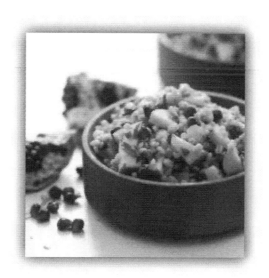

Breakfast Salad from Grains and Fruits

- ➢ Preparation time: 5 minutes
- ➢ Cooking time: 15 minutes
- ➢ Servings: 6
- ➢ Level of difficulty: Easy

Ingredients:

- 1 8-oz low-fat vanilla yogurt

- 1 cup raisins

- 1 orange

- 1 delicious red apple

- 1 Granny Smith apple

- ¾ cup bulgur

- ¾ cup quick-cooking brown rice

- ¼ teaspoon salt

- 3 cups of water

Directions:

1. On high fire, place a large pot and bring water to a boil. Add bulgur and rice. Lower fire to a simmer and cooks for ten minutes while covered.

2. Turn off fire, set aside for 2 minutes while covered. Transfer on a baking sheet, and evenly spread grains to cool.

3. Meanwhile, peel oranges and cut them into sections—chop and core apples. Once grains are cold, transfer to a large serving bowl along with fruits. Add yogurt and mix well to coat. Serve and enjoy.

Nutrition:

Calories: 187

French Toast with Applesauce

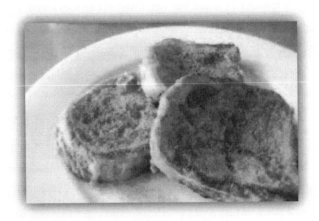

- ➢ Preparation time: 5 minutes
- ➢ Cooking time: 15 minutes
- ➢ Servings: 6

➢ Level of difficulty: Easy

Ingredients:

- ¼ cup unsweetened applesauce

- ½ cup milk

- 1 teaspoon ground cinnamon

- 2 eggs

- 2 tablespoon white sugar

- 6 slices whole-wheat bread

Directions:

1. Mix well applesauce, sugar, cinnamon, milk, and eggs in a mixing bowl. Dip the bread into applesauce mixture until wet; take note that you should do this one slice at a time.

2. On medium fire, heat a nonstick skillet greased with cooking spray. Add soaked bread one at a time and cook for 2-3 minutes per side or until lightly browned. Serve and enjoy.

Nutrition:

Calories: 57

Carbs: 6g

Protein: 4g

Fats: 4g

Bagels Made Healthy

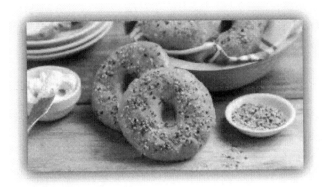

- ➢ Preparation time: 5 minutes
- ➢ Cooking time: 25 minutes
- ➢ Servings: 8
- ➢ Level of difficulty: Normal

Ingredients:

- • 2 teaspoon yeast

- • 1 ½ tablespoon olive oil

- • 1 ¼ cups bread flour

- • 2 cups rice flour

- • 1 tablespoon apple vinegar

- • 2 tablespoon honey

- • 1 ½ cups warm water

- • Seeds to decorate

Directions:

1. In a bread machine, mix all ingredients, and then process on dough cycle. Once done or end of the cycle, create 8 pieces shaped like a flattened ball.

2. Using your thumb, you must create a hole at the center of each, then create a donut shape. Place donut-shaped dough on a greased baking sheet then covers and let it rise for about ½ hour.

3. Prepare about 2 inches of water to boil in a large pan. In boiling water, drop one at a time the bagels and simmer for 1 minute, then turn them once.

4. Remove them and return them to a baking sheet and bake at 350oF (175oC) for about 20 to 25 minutes until golden brown.

Nutrition:

Calories: 221

Carbs: 42g

Protein: 7g

Fats: 5g

Cornbread with Southern Twist

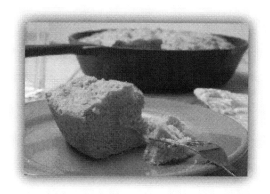

➢ Preparation time: 15 minutes
➢ Cooking time: 60 minutes
➢ Servings: 8
➢ Level of difficulty: Normal

Ingredients:

- 2 teaspoons ghee

- 1 ¼ cups skim milk

- ¼ cup egg white

- 4 tablespoons sodium-free baking powder

- ½ cup rice flour

- 1 ½ cups cornmeal

Directions:

1. Prepare your 8 x 8-inch baking dish or a black iron skillet, then add ghee. Put the baking dish or skillet inside the oven at 425 F; once the ghee has melted, that means the pan is hot already.

2. In a bowl, add milk and egg, then mix well. Take out the skillet and add the melted shortening into the batter and stir well.

3. Pour mixture into skillet after mixing all ingredients. Cook the cornbread for 15-20 minutes until it is golden brown.

Nutrition:

Calories: 166

Carbs: 35 g

Protein: 7 g

Fats: 5 g

Grandma's Pancake Special

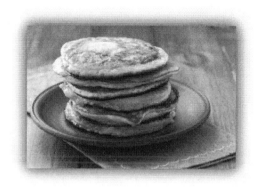

➤ Preparation time: 5 minutes

➤ Cooking time: 15 minutes

➤ Servings: 3

➤ Level of difficulty: Easy

Ingredients:

- 1 tablespoon olive oil

- 1 cup almond milk

- 1 egg

- 2 teaspoons sodium-free baking powder

- 2 tablespoons brown sugar

- 1 ¼ cups flour

Directions:

1. Mix all the dry fixings such as flour, sugar, and baking powder. Mix oil, milk, plus egg in another bowl. Once done, add them all to the flour mixture.

2. Make sure that as you stir the mixture, blend them until slightly lumpy. In a hot, greased griddle, pour-in at least ¼ cup of the batter to make each pancake.

3. To cook, ensure that the bottom is a bit brown, then turn and cook the other side, as well.

Nutrition:

Calories: 167

Carbs: 50 g

Protein: 12 g

Fats: 11 g

Barley with lentil dahl

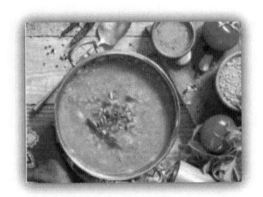

➤ Preparation time: 5 minutes
➤ Cooking time: 35 minutes
➤ Servings: 4
➤ Level of difficulty: Easy

Ingredients:

- ½ cup dried lentils
- ½ cup barley
- 3 cups hot water
- 2 dried red chilies (whole)
- 1 teaspoon turmeric
- 1 teaspoon ground cumin
- 2 cloves garlic

- 2 diced tomatoes
- 1 big onion
- ¼-½ cup fresh cilantro
- 1 tablespoon low-fat sour cream (if desired)

Directions:

1. Rinse the lentils and barley.

2. Prepare a light stir-fry with onion, garlic, and peppers. Combine all other ingredients in the pan except cilantro, add water, and bring to a boil over medium-high heat.

3. Be sure to cover and reduce heat slightly to medium-low and simmer until barley and lentils are tender, about 30 minutes.

4. Next, remove the chiles, then add the cilantro and top with a tablespoon of low-fat sour cream, if desired.

Nutrition:

Calories: 175

Carbs: 40g

Protein: 3g

Fats: 2g

Apple Pumpkin Muffins

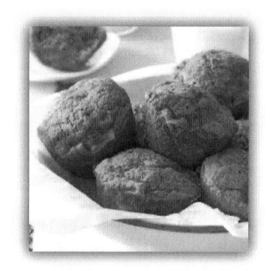

- ➢ Preparation Time: 15 minutes
- ➢ Cooking Time: 20 minutes
- ➢ Servings: 12
- ➢ Level of difficulty: Easy

Ingredients:

- 1 cup kamut flour

- 1 cup wheat bran

- 2 teaspoons Phosphorus Powder

- 1 cup pumpkin purée

- ¼ cup honey

- ¼ cup olive oil

- 1 egg

- 1 teaspoon vanilla extract

- ½ cup cored diced apple

Directions:

1. Preheat the oven to 400°F. Line 12 muffin cups with paper liners. Mix the flour, wheat bran, plus baking powder, mix this in a medium bowl.

2. In a small bowl, whisk the pumpkin, honey, olive oil, egg, plus vanilla. Mix the pumpkin batter into the flour mixture until just combined.

3. Stir in the diced apple. Spoon the batter in the muffin cups. Bake within 20 minutes, or until a toothpick inserted in the center of a muffin comes out clean.

Nutrition:

Calories: 125

Fat: 5g

Carbohydrates: 20g

Protein: 2g

French Toast with Cinnamon and Berries

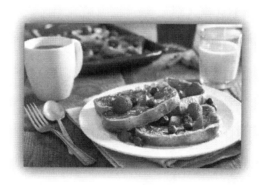

➤ Preparation Time: 15 minutes
➤ Cooking Time: 12 minutes
➤ Servings: 4
➤ Level of difficulty: Easy

Ingredients:

- 4 eggs

- ½ cup rice milk

- ¼ cup freshly squeezed orange juice

- 1 teaspoon ground cinnamon

- ½ teaspoon ground ginger

- pinch ground cloves

- 1 tablespoon ghee (or clarified butter)

- 8 slices whole-grain bread

- 1 cup strawberry and blueberries

Directions:

1. Whisk eggs, rice milk, orange juice, cinnamon, ginger, and cloves until well blended in a large bowl.

2. Dissolve half the ghee in a large skillet. It should be in medium-high heat only.

3. Dredge four of the bread slices in the egg mixture until well soaked, and place them in the skillet. Cook the toast within 6 minutes total.

4. Repeat with the remaining ghee and bread. Serve 2 pieces of hot French toast to each person.

5. Garnish with the strawberries and berries.

Nutrition:

Calories: 236

fat: 11g

Carbohydrates: 27g

Breakfast Tacos

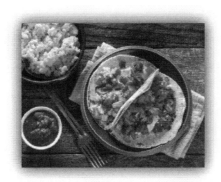

➢ Preparation Time: 10 minutes

➢ Cooking Time: 10 minutes

➢ Servings: 4

➢ Level of difficulty: Easy

Ingredients:

- 1 teaspoon olive oil

- ½ sweet onion, chopped

- ½ red bell pepper, chopped

- ½ teaspoon minced garlic

- 4 eggs, beaten

- ½ teaspoon ground cumin

- Pinch red pepper flakes

- 4 kamut flour tortillas

- ¼ cup tomato salsa

Directions:

1. Chop garlic, onion and peppers.

2. Heat oil in a large skillet over medium heat. Add chopped onion, bell bell pepper and garlic and sauté until softened, about 5 minutes. Add the tomato sauce and cook another 10 minutes.

3. Meanwhile, mix the eggs, cumin and chili in a skillet, and scramble until the eggs are cooked and fluffy. Spoon one-fourth of the egg mixture into the center of each tortilla, and top each with 1 tablespoon of salsa. Serve immediately.

Nutrition:

Calories: 211

Fat: 7g

Carbohydrates: 17g

Protein: 9g

Mexican Scrambled Eggs in Tortilla

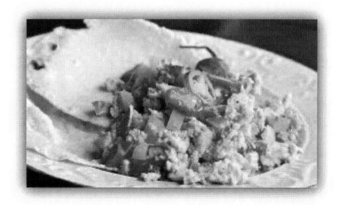

- ➢ Preparation Time: 5 minutes
- ➢ Cooking Time: 2 minutes
- ➢ Servings: 2
- ➢ Level of difficulty: Easy

Ingredients:

- 2 medium corn tortillas

- 4 egg whites

- 1 teaspoon of cumin

- 3 teaspoons of green chilies, diced

- ½ teaspoon of hot pepper sauce

- 2 tablespoons of salsa

- ½ teaspoon whole sea salt

Directions:

1. Spray some olive oil on a medium skillet and heat for a few seconds. Whisk the eggs with the green chilies, hot sauce, and comminute.

2. Add the eggs into the pan, and whisk with a spatula to scramble. Add the salt. Cook until fluffy and done (1-2 minutes) over low heat.

3. Open the tortillas and spread 1 tablespoon of salsa on each. Distribute the egg mixture onto the tortillas and wrap gently to make a burrito. Serve warm.

Nutrition:

Calories: 44.1

Carbohydrate: 2.23 g

Protein: 7.69 g

Fat: 2.39 g

American Blueberry Pancakes

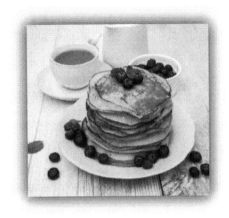

- ➢ Preparation Time: 5 minutes
- ➢ Cooking Time: 10 minutes
- ➢ Servings: 6
- ➢ Level of difficulty: Easy

Ingredients:

- 1 ½ cups of rice flour
- 1 cup of buttermilk
- 2 tablespoons stevia (or 3 tablespoons erythritol)
- 2 tablespoons melted clarified butter or ghee
- 2 teaspoons phosphate-free baking powder
- 2 eggs, beaten
- 1 cup of canned blueberries, rinsed

Directions:

1. Combine the baking powder, flour, and sugar in a bowl. Make a hole in the middle, then slowly add the rest of the ingredients.
2. Begin to stir gently from the sides to the center with a spatula until you get a smooth and creamy batter. With a little ghee, oil the pan and place over medium heat.
3. Take one measuring cup and fill 1/3rd of its capacity with the batter to make each pancake.

4.   Use a spoon to pour the pancake batter and let cook until golden brown. Flip once to cook the other side. Serve warm with optional agave syrup.

Nutrition:

Calories: 238

Carbohydrate: 41.68 g

Protein: 7.2 g

Fat: 6.47 g

Summer Veggie Omelet

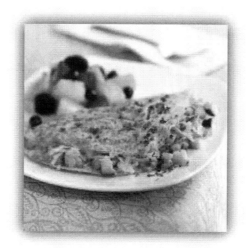

- ➤ Preparation Time: 5 minutes
- ➤ Cooking Time: 5 minutes
- ➤ Servings: 2
- ➤ Level of difficulty: Easy

Ingredients:

- 4 large egg whites
- ¼ cup sweet corn
- 1/2 cup zucchini
- 2 onions
- 2 tablespoons low-fat cream cheese

- 1 pinch black pepper
- 1 pinch chopped parsley

Directions:

1. Chop onions and zucchini.
2. Grease a medium skillet with oil and add the chopped onions, corn and zucchini. Sauté for a couple of minutes until softened. Set half of them aside.
3. Beat the eggs with the water, 1 tablespoon of the cream cheese and the pepper in a bowl. Add the eggs to the vegetable mixture in the skillet. Allow to cook, moving the edges with a spatula to allow the raw egg to cook evenly.
4. Flip the omelet with the help of a plate. Place on top of the pan and flip, then back into the pan. Pour over half of the remaining vegetables and the tablespoon of cream cheese. Let stand for another 1-2 minutes. Fold in half and serve. Decorate with parsley.

Calories: 90

Carbohydrates: 15.97 g

Protein: 8.07 g

Fats: 2.44 g

Raspberry Overnight Porridge

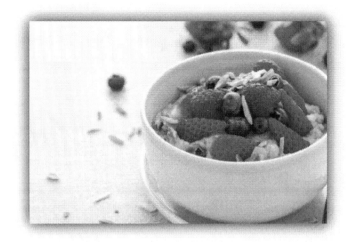

- ➢ Preparation Time: Overnight
- ➢ Cooking Time: 0 minute
- ➢ Servings:12
- ➢ Level of difficulty: Easy

Ingredients:

- ½ cup oatmeal

- ½ cup almond milk

- 1 tablespoon of honey

- 5-6 raspberries, fresh

- ½ cup berries and strawberries, fresh or frozen

- 1 tablespoon almond flakes

Directions:

1. Combine the oats, almond milk, and honey in a mason jar and place into the fridge overnight. Serve the next morning with berries and strawberries, and the almond flakes on top.

Nutrition:

Calories: 143.6

Carbohydrate: 34.62 g

Protein: 3.44 g

Fat: 3.91 g

Cheesy Scrambled Eggs with Fresh Herbs

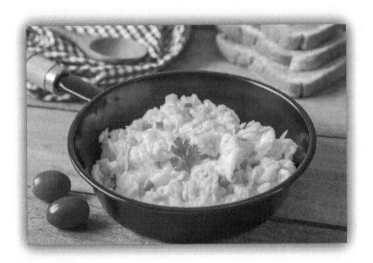

- ➢ Preparation Time: 15 minutes
- ➢ Cooking Time: 10 minutes
- ➢ Servings: 4
- ➢ Level of difficulty: Easy

Ingredients:

- 3 eggs

- 2 egg whites

- ½ cup cream cheese

- ¼ cup unsweetened rice milk

- 1 tbsp chopped scallion, green part only

- 1 tbsp chopped fresh tarragon

- 2 tbsp grass-fed unsalted butter

- ground black pepper to taste

Directions:

1. In a container, mix the eggs, egg whites, cream cheese, rice milk, scallions, and tarragon until mixed and smooth. Melt the butter in a skillet.

2. Pour in the egg mix and cook, stirring, for 5 minutes or until the eggs are thick and curds creamy. Season with pepper and serve.

Nutrition:

Calories: 221

Fat: 19g

Carb: 3g

Protein: 8g

Turkey and Spinach Omelette

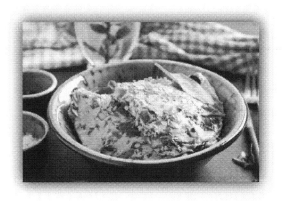

➢ Preparation Time: 2 minutes
➢ Cooking Time: 14 minutes
➢ Servings: 2

> Level of difficulty: Easy

Ingredients:

- 4 eggs
- 1 tsp extra virgin olive oil
- 1 cup raw spinach
- ½ garlic, minced
- 1 tsp nutmeg, grated
- 1 cup cooked and diced turkey breast
- 1 pinch of pepper
- 1 handful of parsley 1 tsp balsamic vinegar

Directions:

1. Heat a pot over a source of heat and add oil. Add turkey and heat through for 6 to 8 minutes. Add spinach, garlic, and nutmeg and stir-fry for 6 minutes more.
2. Beat the eggs in a dish and pour the mixture over the turkey in the pan. Wait a couple of minutes, fold the omelet over and turn it on its side.
3. Serve hot with pepper and parsley.

Nutrition:

Calories: 301

Fat: 19g

Carb: 12g

Protein: 19g

Mexican Style Burritos

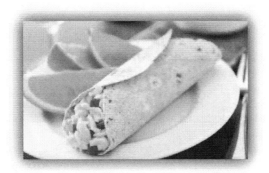

> ➤ Preparation Time: 5 minutes
> ➤ Cooking Time: 15 minutes
> ➤ Servings: 2
> ➤ Level of difficulty: Easy

Ingredients:

- 1 tbsp olive oil

- 2 corn tortillas

- ¼ cup red onion, chopped

- ¼ cup red bell peppers, chopped

- ½ red chili, deseeded and chopped

- 2 eggs

- 1 lime, juiced

- 1 tbsp cilantro, chopped

Directions:

1. Turn the broiler to medium heat. Place the tortillas underneath for 1 to 2 minutes on each side or until lightly toasted. Remove and keep the broiler on.

2. Sauté onion, chili, and bell peppers for 5 to 6 minutes or until soft. Place the eggs on top of the onions and peppers. Place skillet under the broiler for 5-6 minutes or until the eggs are cooked.

3. Serve half the eggs and vegetables on top of each tortilla and sprinkle with cilantro and lime juice to serve.

Nutrition:

Calories: 202

Fat: 13g

Carb: 19g

Protein: 9g

Rye flour Pancakes

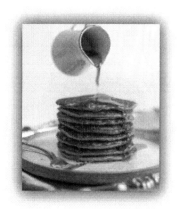

- ➢ Preparation Time: 10 minutes
- ➢ Cooking Time: 5 minutes
- ➢ Servings: 5
- ➢ Level of difficulty: Easy

Ingredients:

- 1 cup rye flour

- 1 tbsp erythritol (or sweetener as needed)

- 2 tsp phosphate-free baking powder

- 2 egg whites

- 1 cup almond milk

- 2 tbsp olive oil

- 1 tbsp maple extract

Directions:

1. Mix the flour, sweetener, plus baking powder in a bowl. Make a well or a hole in the center and place to one side. Mix the egg whites, milk, oil, and maple extract, do this in another bowl.

2. Add the egg mixture to the well and gently mix until a batter is formed—heat skillet over medium heat.

3. Cook within 2 minutes on each side or until the pancake is golden; add 1/5 of the batter to the pan. Repeat with the remaining batter and serve.

Nutrition:

Calories: 178

Fat: 3 g

Protein: 6 g

Carb: 4 g

Buckwheat and Grapefruit Porridge

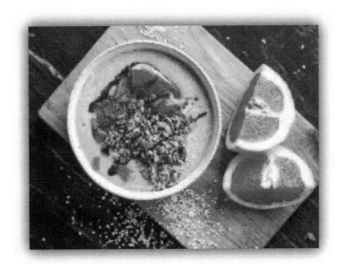

- ➢ Preparation Time: 5 minutes
- ➢ Cooking Time: 20 minutes
- ➢ Servings: 2
- ➢ Level of difficulty: Easy

Ingredients:

- ½ cup Buckwheat

- ¼ grapefruit, chopped

- 1 tbsp Honey

- 1 ½ cup Almond milk

- 2 cups of water

Directions:

1. Boil water on the stove. Add the buckwheat and place the lid on the pan. Simmer for 7 to 10 minutes in low heat. Check to ensure water does not dry out.

2. Remove and set aside for 5 minutes, do this when most of the water is absorbed. Drain excess water from the pan and stir in almond milk, heating through for 5 minutes. Add the honey and grapefruit. Serve.

Nutrition:

Calories: 231

Fat: 4 g

Carb: 43 g

Protein: 2 g

Egg and Veggie Muffins

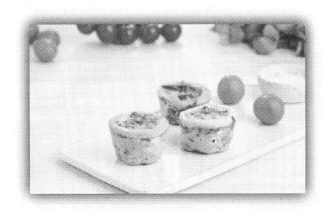

- ➢ Preparation Time: 15 minutes
- ➢ Cooking Time: 20 minutes
- ➢ Servings: 4
- ➢ Level of difficulty: Easy

Ingredients:

- Olive oil for the muffin pans

- 4 eggs

- 2 tbsp unsweetened rice milk

- ½ sweet onion, chopped

- ½ red bell pepper, chopped

- pinch red pepper flakes
- pinch ground black pepper

Directions:

1. Preheat the oven to 350F. Oil 4 muffin pans with olive oil. Set aside. Whisk together the milk, eggs, onion, red pepper, parsley, red pepper flakes, and black pepper until mixed.

2. Pour the egg mixture into prepared muffin pans. Bake until the muffins are puffed and golden, about 18 to 20 minutes. Serve

Nutrition:

Calories: 84

Fat: 5g

Carb: 3g

Protein: 7g

Festive Berry Parfait

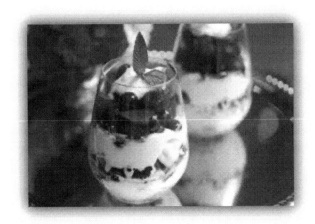

- ➢ Preparation Time: 20 minutes
- ➢ Cooking Time: 0 minutes
- ➢ Servings: 4
- ➢ Level of difficulty: Easy

Ingredients:

- 1 cup vanilla rice milk, at room temperature
- ½ cup plain cream cheese, room temperature
- 1 tbsp brown sugar
- ½ tsp ground cinnamon
- 1 cup crumbled meringue cookies
- 2 cups fresh blueberries
- 1 cup sliced fresh strawberries

Directions:

1. Mix the milk, cream cheese, sugar, and cinnamon in a small bowl until smooth. Into 4 (6-ounce) glasses, spoon ¼ cup of crumbled cookie in the bottom of each.

2. Spoon ¼ cup of the cream cheese mixture on top of the cookies. Top the cream cheese with ¼ cup of the berries.

3. Repeat in each cup with the cookies, cream cheese mixture, and berries. Chill in the refrigerator for 1 hour and serve.

Nutrition:

Calories: 243

Fat: 1 g

Carbs: 33 g

Protein: 4 g

Simple Chia Porridge

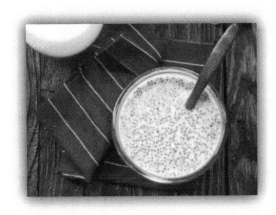

- ➤ Preparation Time: 10 minutes
- ➤ Cooking Time: 5-10 minutes
- ➤ Servings: 2
- ➤ Level of difficulty: Easy

Ingredients:

- 1 tablespoon chia seeds
- 1 tablespoon ground flaxseed
- 1/3 cup coconut cream
- ½ cup of water
- 1 teaspoon vanilla extract
- 1 tablespoon almond butter

Directions:

1. Add chia seeds, coconut cream, flaxseed, water, and vanilla to a small pot. Stir and let it sit within 5 minutes. Add almond butter and place pot over low heat.

2. Keep stirring as almond butter melts. Once the porridge is hot/not boiling, pour into a bowl. Add a few berries or a dash of cream for extra flavor.

Nutrition:

Calories: 310

Fat: 38g

Carbohydrates: 10g

Protein: 6g

Berry Salad with Italian Ricotta Cheese

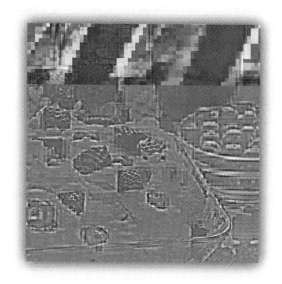

- ➤ Preparation Time: 5 minutes
- ➤ Cooking time: 0 minutes
- ➤ Servings: 2
- ➤ Level of difficulty: Easy

Ingredients:

- 1 cup fresh blackberries, sliced

- 1 cup fresh blueberries, sliced

- 2 cups fresh strawberries, sliced

- 1/3 cup lemon juice

- 2 cups fresh Italian ricotta cheese

- 1/8 tsp. Cinnamon

Directions:

1. Mix all berries in a bowl, set aside. Add some lemon juice from the cup. Put the ricotta cheese on a round plate or a bowl, and then cover it with berries. Spread the cinnamon on it.
2. Top with the berries, a pinch of cinnamon, and serve.

Nutrition:

Calories: 140

Protein: 15 g

Carbs: 23g

Fat: 12g

Rhubarb Bread Pudding

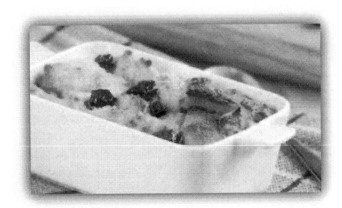

➤ Preparation Time: 15 minutes
➤ Cooking Time: 50 minutes
➤ Servings: 6
➤ Level of difficulty: Normal

Ingredients:

- unsalted butter, for greasing the baking dish
- 1 ½ cup unsweetened rice milk
- 3 eggs
- ½ cup brown sugar
- 1 tbsp cornstarch
- 1 vanilla bean, split
- 10 10 slices of stale bread without salt, cut into 1-inch chunks
- 2 cups chopped fresh rhubarb

Directions:

1. Warm oven to 350 F. Oiled an 8-by-8-inch baking dish with butter. Set aside. Mix the eggs, rice milk, sugar, and cornstarch in a bowl.

2. Scrape the vanilla seeds into the milk batter, then whisk to blend. Put the bread in the egg batter and stir to coat the bread thoroughly. Put the chopped rhubarb and mix.

3. Let the bread and egg mixture soak within 30 minutes. Spoon the batter into your prepared baking dish, cover with aluminum foil, and bake for 40 minutes.

4. Uncover the bread pudding and bake for 10 minutes more or until the pudding is golden brown and set. Serve warm.

Nutrition:

Calories: 197

Fat: 4 g

Carbs: 3 g

Protein: 6 g

Fruit and Cheese Breakfast Wrap

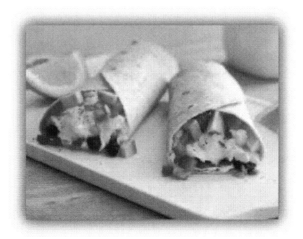

- ➢ Preparation Time: 10 minutes
- ➢ Cooking Time: 0 minutes
- ➢ Servings: 2
- ➢ Level of difficulty: Easy

Ingredients:

- 2 flour tortillas

- 2 tbsp plain cream cheese

- 1 apple, peeled, cored, and sliced thinly

- 1 tbsp honey

Directions:

1. Put both tortillas on a clean surface, then spread 1 tbsp of cream cheese, leaving about ½ inch around its edges.

2. Put the apple slices on the cream cheese. Drizzle honey on the apples lightly. Fold both left plus right edges of the tortillas into the center.

3. Fold it on the fruit and the side pieces. Roll the tortilla away from you, creating a snug wrap. Repeat with the second tortilla, then serve.

Nutrition:

Calories: 188

Fat: 6 g

Carbs: 33 g

Protein: 4 g

Hot Breakfast Burrito

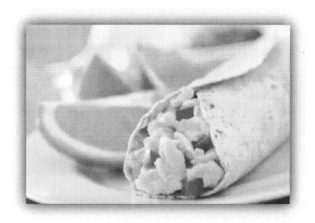

➢ Preparation Time: 5 minutes
➢ Cooking Time: 5 minutes
➢ Servings: 2
➢ Level of difficulty: Easy

Ingredients:

- 4 eggs

- 3 tbsp. Ortega green chilies, diced

- 2 flour tortillas, Burrito size

- Olive oil for pan

- ¼ tsp. ground cumin

- ½ tsp. hot pepper sauce

Directions:

1. Oiled a skillet using olive oil and heat over medium heat. Beat the eggs with the green chilies, cumin, and hot sauce.

2. Pour the eggs into the skillet and cook for 1 to 2 minutes until set. Warm-up the tortillas for a few seconds in the microwave until they are warm. Place half the egg mixture onto each tortilla and roll up burrito style.

Nutrition:

Calories: 366

Carbs: 33g

Fat: 0 g

Protein: 22g

Baked Frittata with lean meat

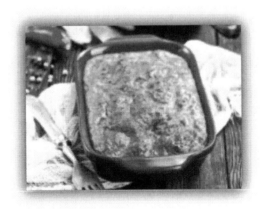

- ➢ Preparation Time: 15 minutes
- ➢ Cooking Time: 1 hour
- ➢ Servings: 9
- ➢ Level of difficulty: Normal

Ingredients:

- • 8 oz reduced-fat meat, crumbled

- 1 cup cream cheese

- 1 cup 1% low-fat milk

- 4 slices white bread, cubed or broken

- 5 large eggs

- ½ tsp. dry mustard

- ½ tsp. dried onion flakes

Directions:

1. Preheat oven to 325 F. Grease a baking dish. Brown ground beef in a skillet and set aside.
2. Separate the egg yolks from the egg whites and whip the latter.
3. Mix the cream cheese, egg yolks and milk in a mixer.
4. Pour the chopped meat into the egg mixture. Carefully add the beaten egg whites.
5. Pour the egg and meat mixture into the baking dish. Bake 50 minutes or until mixture is golden brown. Cut into 9 servings and serve.

Nutrition:

Calories: 223

Carbs: 12g

Protein: 10g

Fat: 9 g

Buckwheat Breakfast Bowl

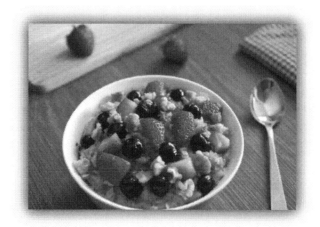

- ➢ Preparation Time: 20 minutes
- ➢ Cooking Time: 20 minutes
- ➢ Servings: 4
- ➢ Level of difficulty: Normal

Ingredients:

- ½ cup buckwheat grains, uncooked

- 1 medium fresh pear, thinly sliced

- 1 tbsp. ghee

- 1 cup fresh cranberries and strawberries

- 1 tsp. fresh orange zest

- 2 tbsp maple syrup

- ½ tsp. cinnamon

- grated ginger root

Directions:

1. Cook the buckwheat grains,s in 1½ cups of water. Bring to a boil and simmer for 20 minutes. Check the cooking point and bake for another 10 minutes or so if needed (it should remain crunchy).

2. Sauté the pears in the ghee until soft. Add the cranberries, strawberries and ginger and cook until the berries burst. Add buckwheat, orange zest, maple syrup, and cinnamon and serve.

Nutrition:

Calories: 174

Carbs: 36g

Protein: 3g

Fat: 2,5 g

Breakfast Toast

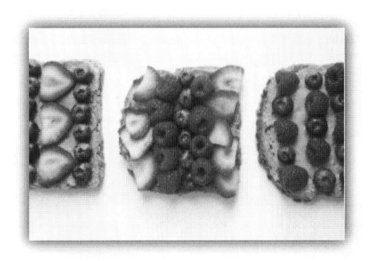

- ➤ Preparation Time: 10 minutes
- ➤ Cooking Time: 10 minutes
- ➤ Servings: 2
- ➤ Level of difficulty: Easy

Ingredients:

- strawberries, blueberries and raspberries
- slices of whole grain bread
- 1 tablespoon of creamy, unsalted natural peanut butter 6 strawberries, sliced

Directions:

1. Toast the bread. Spread the bread with peanut butter. Top with the berries and serve.

Nutrition:

Calories: 290

Carbs: 45g

Fat 25 g

Protein: 10g

Asparagus Cauliflower Tortilla

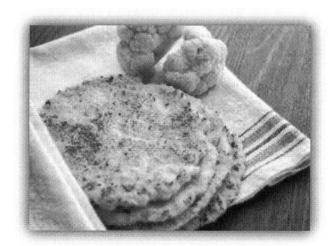

➢ Preparation Time: 15 minutes
➢ Cooking Time: 15 minutes
➢ Servings: 4
➢ Level of difficulty: Normal

Ingredients:

*   2 cup asparagus, chopped into bite-size pieces

*   2 cup cauliflower, chopped into bite-size pieces

- 1½ cup onion, finely chopped

- 3 eggs

- 2 tbsp. fresh parsley, finely chopped

- 2 tsp. olive oil

- Salt and freshly ground pepper

- ¼ tsp. dried thyme

- ¼ tsp. ground nutmeg

- ¼ teaspoon of dried thyme

- 1 garlic clove, minced

Directions:

1. Place the asparagus and cauliflower in a dish with 1 tablespoon of water. Cook on high for around 3 to 5 minutes until tender but also crisp.
2. Sauté the onion in a skillet until translucent. Stir in the vegetables and remaining ingredients, and reduce the heat.
3. Cook within 10 to 15 minutes or until set and brown around the edges. Use a spatula to slide the tortilla onto a warm platter or serving plate. Slice into wedges and serve—also, delicious cold or reheated.

Nutrition:

Calories: 102

Carbs: 5g

Fat: 0g

Protein: 9g

French Toast with honey and cinnamon

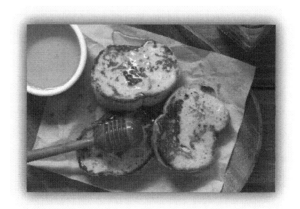

- ➢ Preparation Time: 15 minutes
- ➢ Cooking Time: 15 minutes
- ➢ Servings: 4
- ➢ Level of difficulty: Easy

Ingredients:

- 4 slices of salt-free bread

- 4 cup rice milk, non-enriched

- 4 eggs

- 4 tbsp. ghee

- ½ cup Erythritol (or other sweetener)

- 1 tsp. cinnamon

- 1 tsp. honey

- Ghee for the pan

Directions:

1. Melt ghee in nonstick pan. Lightly roast bread slices in it.
2. Beat the eggs, rice milk, erythritol and cinnamon and dip the bread slices in it.
3. Bake for 40-50 minutes in a preheated 350 F oven, then serve warm and drizzled with honey.

Nutrition:

Calories: 450

Carbs: 65g

Fat: 2g

Protein: 16g

Lunch Recipes: healthy, easy, and tasty dishes

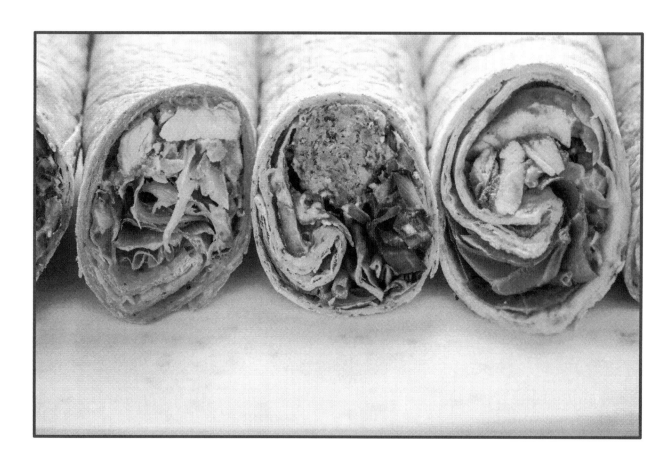

Herbed veal meatloaf

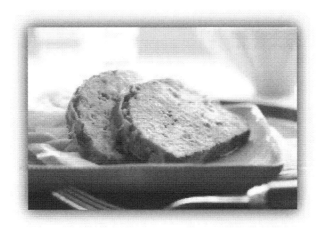

- ➢ Preparation Time: 10 minutes
- ➢ Cooking time: 50 minutes
- ➢ Servings: 8
- ➢ Level of difficulty: Normal

Ingredients:

- 1 lb. lean ground veal

- ½ cup breadcrumbs

- ½ cup chopped sweet onion

- 1 egg

- tablespoons fresh chopped basil

- 1 teaspoon fresh chopped thyme

- 1 teaspoon fresh chopped parsley

- ¼ teaspoon ground black pepper

- 1 tablespoon brown sugar

- 1 tablespoon apple cider vinegar

- ¼ teaspoon garlic powder

Directions:

1. Preheat oven to 400°F. Mix the breadcrumbs, meat, onion, basil, egg, thyme, parsley, plus pepper until well combined.
2. Place the meat in a rectangular shaped baking dish. Mix brown sugar, apple cider vinegar, and garlic powder in a small bowl.
3. Spread the emulsion evenly over the meat. Bake the meatloaf for about 50 minutes, check according to oven type. Let rest for 10 minutes and then discard any excess fat. Let it warm and then serve.

Nutrition:

Calories: 220

Protein: 24 g

Carbs: 4g

Fat: 13g

Roast-beef Wraps

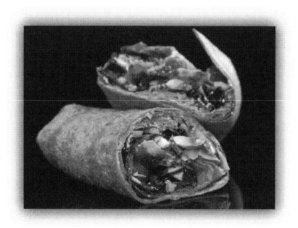

- ➢ Preparation Time: 10 minutes
- ➢ Cooking time: 0 minutes
- ➢ Servings: 2

➢ Level of difficulty: Easy

Ingredients:

- 50 gr red radish
- 2 whole wheat flour tortillas
- 2 tablespoons low-fat quark cheese
- 1/4 bowl chopped red onion
- 1/4 cup sweet bell pepper cut into strips
- 1 tbsp blended herb dressing (parsley, oil, lemon, salt, pepper, garlic)

Directions:

1. Spread quark over the surface of the wrap. Use ingredients to make two wraps. Layer tortillas with roast beef, onions, arugula, champignons, bell pepper, and radish.
2. Sprinkle with the herb seasoning. Roll up wraps and cut into two pieces each. Serve fresh.

Calories: 255

Protein: 24g

Carbs: 20g

Fats: 3g

Salmon and rice wraps

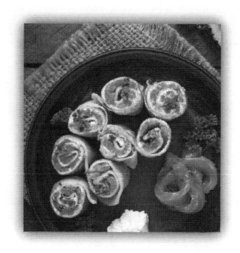

- ➢ Preparation Time: 10 minutes
- ➢ Cooking time: 10 minutes
- ➢ Servings: 2
- ➢ Level of difficulty: Normal

Ingredients:

- 2 whole eggs
- 7 oz rice flour
- ½ cup water
- Oil for pan
- 7 oz wild smoked salmon
- 2 oz spreadable fresh cheese
- parsley

Directions:

1 Beat the eggs with the rice flour and water, creating a smooth batter.

2 Heat a pan of about 8 inches with a drizzle of oil and pour the batter distributing it on the bottom, trying to make a homogeneous shape and round.

3 Once ready, spread the cream cheese on the surface, distribute the salmon slices, a little parsley, and roll up.

Nutrition:

Calories: 223

Protein: 15g

Carbs: 24g

Fats: 20g

Chicken Salad

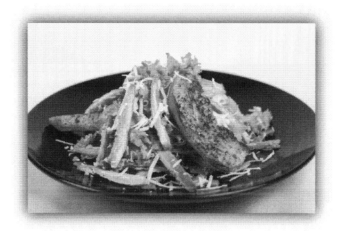

➢ Preparation Time: 10 minutes

➢ Cooking time: 0 minutes

➢ Servings: 2

➢ Level of difficulty: Easy

Ingredients:

- 7 oz of chicken breast
- 5 oz mixed salad
- 4 slices of bread without salt
- Parmesan cheese in flakes
- Apple vinegar
- ½ lemon
- Extra virgin olive oil1 tbsp. onion, chopped

Directions:

1. Cut the chicken breast and roast it in a nonstick skillet.
2. Wash the salad and distribute in a bowl or serving dish.
3. Spread the chicken cut into strips on top and dress with a vinaigrette of oil, lemon and apple cider vinegar.
4. Sprinkle with shredded Parmesan cheese and serve. Put everything in the bagel on the lettuce leaves, adding some mayonnaise, and then close the bread. Serve and enjoy!

Nutrition:

Calories: 245

Protein: 22 g

Carbs: 24 g

Fat: 8 g

Tuna and asparagus salad

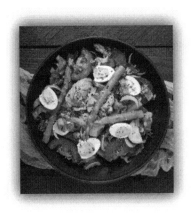

➤ Preparation Time: 10 minutes
➤ Cooking time: 15 minutes
➤ Servings: 2
➤ Level of difficulty: Easy

Ingredients:

- 1 package of low-sodium tuna, cut into small pieces
- 5 oz of asparagus
- 2 eggs
- 1 fresh tomato
- ½ red onion
- Mixed salad
- 1 tablespoon of extra virgin olive oil
- pepper

- lemon

Directions:

1. Boil the asparagus for 20 minutes and use the softer part
2. Harden the eggs and let them cool
3. Mix all ingredients in a large bowl, drizzle with oil, pepper, a squeeze of lemon and serve.

Calories: 230

Tiny Rice Pies

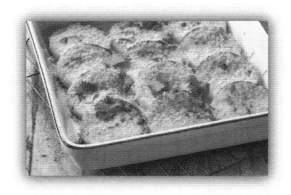

- ➤ Preparation Time: 10 minutes
- ➤ Cooking time: 15 minutes
- ➤ Servings: 2
- ➤ Level of difficulty: Normal

Ingredients:

- ½ cup of rice semolina
- ½ cup cornmeal
- A pinch of whole grain sea salt
- A pinch of pepper
- ¼ cup Greek yogurt
- ¼ cup vegetable broth
- 4 oz. of tofu
- 2 tablespoons grated Parmesan cheese

- A few sprigs of finely chopped parsley
- 1 tbsp. of ghee

Directions:

1. Heat oil in frying pan the semolina, salt. Cook until semolina turns a little brown. Let cool.

2. Combine Greek yogurt with a little water and mix until smooth.

3. Add the cornmeal, pepper, crumbled tofu and mix everything into the semolina, setting aside for 10-15 minutes so it sets.

4. Create round shapes with a pasta cup or other.

5. Put the ghee in a baking dish, arrange the semolina circles and sprinkle with Parmesan cheese.

6. Bake under the broiler for 10 to 15 minutes. Put a little parsley on the semolina circles and serve while still hot.

Nutrition:

Calories: 175

Protein: 5 g

Carbs: 35g

Fat: 12g

Roasted bread with creamy mustard eggs

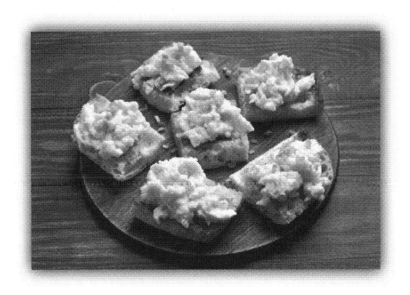

- ➢ Preparation Time: 15 minutes
- ➢ Cooking time: 10 minutes
- ➢ Servings: 2
- ➢ Level of difficulty: Normal

Ingredients:

- 4 slices of stale bread without salt
- 6 eggs
- 4 oz of low-fat quark
- 2 teaspoons of ghee
- ½ cup unsweetened almond milk
- 1/2 tablespoon of mustard

Directions:

1. Toast slices of stale bread and set aside
2. Melt the ghee in a pan and add the eggs with the quark, almond milk and mustard

3. Stir continuously, they must remain creamy.

4. Pour egg mixture over toast before serving.

Nutrition:

Calories: 430

Protein: 15 g

Carbs: 34g

Fat: 21g

Stuffed Peppers

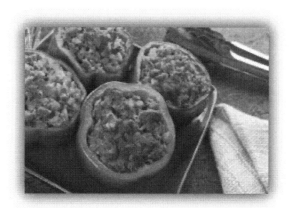

➢ Preparation Time: 10 minutes

➢ Cooking Time: 1 hour and 20 minutes

➢ Servings: 4

➢ Level of difficulty: Normal

Ingredients:

- ¾ pound ground beef
- ½ cup white onion, chopped
- 4 medium green bell peppers, destemmed and cored
- 1 tablespoon dried parsley
- 1 ½ teaspoon garlic powder
- 1 teaspoon ground black pepper
- 2 cups cooked white rice

- 3 ounces tomato sauce, unsalted

Directions:

1. Switch on the oven, then set it to 375 F and let it preheat. Take a medium-sized saucepan, place it over medium heat and when hot, add beef and cook for 10 minutes, or until browned.

2. Then drain the excess fat, add remaining ingredients (except for green bell pepper), stir until combined, and simmer for 10 minutes until cooked.

3. When done, spoon the beef mixture evenly between peppers, place the peppers into a baking dish, and bake for 1 hour until cooked. Serve straight away.

Nutrition:

Calories 264

Fat 7 g

Protein 20 g

Carbohydrates 28 g

Celery Tuna Salad

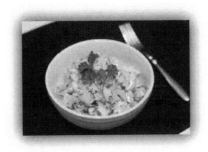

- ➢ Preparation Time: 5 minutes
- ➢ Cooking time: 0 minutes
- ➢ Servings: 2
- ➢ Level of difficulty: Easy

Ingredients:

- 1-piece celery, sliced
- 15 oz. Packed and unsalted tuna
- 1/2 apple, sliced
- 1/2 small onion, chopped
- 2 tbsp. mustard
- 1 tbsp. fresh lemon juice
- A bit of black pepper
- Pinch whole sea salt

Directions:

1. Mix all together, adding mustard, black pepper, and, if you wish, some salt.

Nutrition:

Calories: 20

Protein: 15 g

Carbs: 0g

Fat: 3g

Meat Casserole

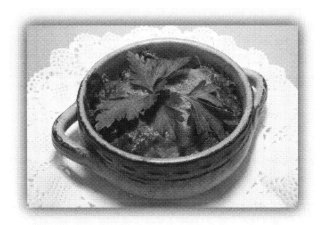

> ➤ Preparation Time: 10 minutes
> ➤ Cooking time: 60 minutes
> ➤ Servings: 10
> ➤ Level of difficulty: Normal

Ingredients:

- 8 oz. lean veal ground meat

- 8 oz. Reduced-fat pork sausage

- 7 oz. Cream cheese

- 1 low-fat glass milk

- 5 eggs

- 1/2 tsp. Dry mustard

- 1 onion

Directions:

1. Preheat oven at 325°f (160°c).

2. Lightly sauté the onion.

3. Cut the sausage and the veal and pour over the sauteed mixture. Set aside and meanwhile mix all other ingredients.

4. Add cooked meat to mixture, pour into earthenware or ovenproof pot and bake for 50 minutes. Cut into 10 portions and serve. Enjoy!

Nutrition:

Calories: 222

Protein: 10 g

Carbs: 3g

Fat: 19g

Ground Beef in A Cup

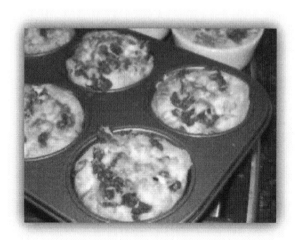

➢ Preparation Time: 10 minutes
➢ Cooking time: 3 minutes
➢ Servings: 2
➢ Level of difficulty: Easy

Ingredients:

- 1/4-pound ground beef
- 2 tbsp. low-fat milk
- 4 eggs
- 2 tbsp. oatmeal

- 1 onion, finely chopped

Directions:

1. Sauté the onion in very little olive oil and as soon as it cooks, pour in the ground beef.
2. Oil the muffin tins.
3. Beat the eggs in a bowl and make them fluffy.
4. Add the milk and oats.
5. Pour the meat into the bowl and mix everything together.
6. Pour the mixture into the muffin tins and bake at 375F for 20 minutes.

Nutrition:

Calories: 250

Protein: 25 g

Carbs: 1g

Fat: 29g

Spiced turkey breast with vegetables

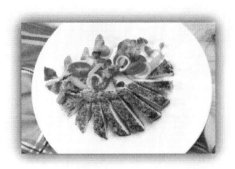

- ➢ Preparation time: 15 minutes
- ➢ Cooking time: 15 minutes
- ➢ Servings: 2
- ➢ Level of difficulty: Easy

Ingredients:

- 300 gr turkey breast
- 1 tbsp dehydrated mixed spices (paprika, turmeric, black pepper, oregano..)
- 5 oz valerian salad
- ½ bell pepper
- ½ cup of cherry tomatoes
- Extra virgin olive oil to taste
- A pinch of salt

Directions:

1. Sprinkle the turkey breast with the spices and a little olive oil and let stand 10 minutes.
2. Wash the vegetables, cut the tomatoes and bell bell pepper into strips
3. Heat a non-stick griddle or frying pan and when hot, place the turkey on it.
4. Cook on both sides until well browned, being careful not to burn it.
5. Place in a serving dish, cut the turkey into slices, surround with the sliced vegetables and season with a drizzle of extra virgin olive oil and a pinch of salt.

Nutrition:

Calories 215

Protein 29 g

Carb. 2.51 g

Fats 12.70 g

Baked Mushrooms with Pumpkin and Polenta

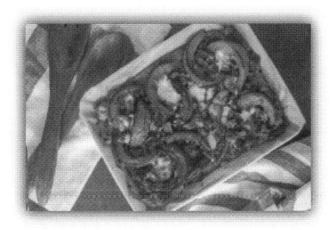

- ➢ Preparation time: 15 minutes
- ➢ Cooking time: 40 minutes
- ➢ Servings: 3
- ➢ Level of difficulty: Normal

Ingredients:

- 900 g mix of mushrooms, chopped
- 9 slices pumpkin
- 1 cup cooked pumpkin puree
- 1/3 cup of EVO oil
- 1 garlic head, crushed cloves
- A small handful of sage, finely chopped or sliced
- Sea salt and freshly ground black pepper
- 3 cups veg broth
- Nutmeg, freshly grated
- 1 chipotle adobo sauce, seedless and finely chopped, plus a small spoon of adobo sauce
- 1 cup quick-cooking polenta
- 1 tbsp ghee
- Chives, minced, for decoration

Directions:

1. Warm your oven to 220 C. Mix the mushrooms with extra virgin olive oil, garlic, brine, salt, plus pepper and bake within 25 minutes.

2. Meanwhile, in a small pan, put it pumpkin puree over medium heat, along with some chicken broth to dilute—season with salt, pepper, and nutmeg.

3. Put the remaining stock and bring to a boil in another pan, then add the polenta, and mix using a wire whisk.

4. Continue beating the polenta until the sides are far from the pan walls, then add the ghee, and beat again.

5. Combine pumpkin and polenta and serve in individual shallow bowls. Top with roasted mushrooms and chives for garnish.

Nutrition:

Calories 151

Protein 7.1 g

Carbs 6.7 g

Fat 10.9 g

Quinoa Salad with Chickpeas and Feta

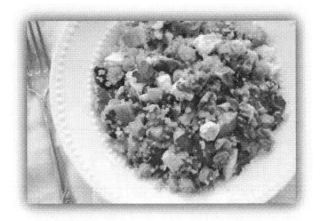

- ➤ Preparation time: 15 minutes
- ➤ Cooking time: 15 minutes
- ➤ Servings: 4
- ➤ Level of difficulty: Normal

Ingredients:

- 1 onion, chopped
- 1 toe garlic, chopped
- 1 tbsp olive oil
- 150 ml vegetable broth
- 100 g Quinoa
- 60 g Feta
- 215 g (Drained weight, from the jar) chickpeas
- 1 small bunch of coriander
- 1/2 lemon
- Salt
- Pepper
- 1/2 tsp Ras el Hanout

Directions:

1. Sauté onion plus garlic in a saucepan with oil. Deglaze using the vegetable stock, bring to the boil and cook the quinoa according to the instructions on the packet.

2. In the meantime, pour the chickpeas out of the glass into a sieve, rinse and drain. Wash the coriander, shake dry and chop.
3. Squeeze the lemon. Prepare a dressing from lemon juice, salt, pepper, Ras el Hanout, and coriander.
4. Put the finished quinoa in a bowl, pour the drained chickpeas and the dressing over it.
5. Finally, crumble the feta and mix it with the quinoa salad. Let it steep for at least 15 minutes. The salad tastes lukewarm or cold.

Nutrition:

Calories 369

Protein 20 g

Fat 20 g

Carbohydrates 52 g

Chicken and Asparagus Salad with Watercress

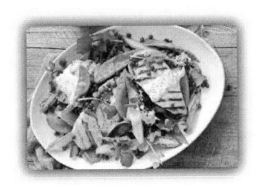

➢ Preparation time: 15 minutes
➢ Cooking time: 5 minutes
➢ Servings: 4
➢ Level of difficulty: Normal

Ingredients:

• 100 g spring onions, cut into thin rings
• 200 g Edamame, boiled

- 100 g green asparagus, thin slices
- 600 g chicken breast fillet (4 chicken breast fillets)
- A pinch of whole sea salt
- A pinch of pepper
- 1 small lime
- 1 clove of garlic
- 3 tbsp honey
- 1 tbsp grainy mustard
- 5 tbsp olive oil
- 100 g watercress

Directions:

1. Wash the chicken fillets, pat dry with kitchen paper, and cut into strips. Season with salt and pepper. For the dressing, cut the lime in half and squeeze out the juice.
2. Peel and dice the garlic. Mix with honey, mustard, 3 tablespoons of lime juice, and 3 tablespoons of oil—season with salt and pepper. Warm-up the rest of the oil in a large non-stick pan and stir-fry the meat for about 5 minutes over high heat.
3. Put the chicken, spring onions, edamame, and asparagus in a bowl. Mix in the dressing and let the salad steep for about 10 minutes.
4. In the meantime, wash the watercress and shake dry. Pluck the leaves, coarsely chop as desired, and distribute on plates or bowls. Flavor the chicken salad with salt and pepper and serve on the cress.

Nutrition:

Calories 185

Protein 37 g

Fat 14 g

Carbohydrates 22 g

Chicken and Zucchini Salad with Nuts

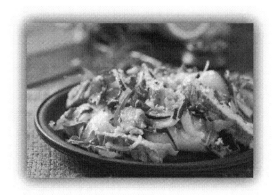

- ➢ Preparation time: 15 minutes
- ➢ Cooking time: 15 minutes
- ➢ Servings: 4
- ➢ Level of difficulty: Normal

Ingredients:

- 3 zucchini cut into strips
- 16 oz chicken breast fillets
- 8 oz of arugula
- salt
- pepper
- 4 tablespoons olive oil
- ½ mint
- ½ lemon
- 80 g walnuts

Directions:

1. Wash the arugula and dry it.
2. Season the zucchini with salt and pepper. Rinse the chicken fillet under cold water and pat dry.
3. In a skillet, heat 2 tablespoons of oil. Brown the chicken in it for about 10 minutes over medium heat until golden brown. Reduce the heat and let the fillets cook.

4. In another skillet, heat the remaining oil. Sauté the zucchini slices for about 4 minutes over medium heat.

5. Wash the mint, shake off the dried leaves, and trim them. Squeeze the lemons in half. Remove the chicken from the pan, drain on paper towels and cut into thin slices.

6. Chop the walnuts coarsely and mix well with the zucchini, chicken, arugula, mint and lemon juice. Season with salt and pepper and arrange in bowls.

Veal Kidneys

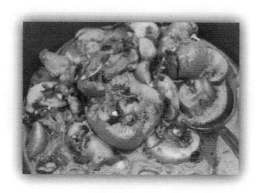

➢ Preparation time: 45 minutes

➢ Cooking time: 10 minutes

➢ Servings: 4

➢ Level of difficulty: Normal

Ingredients:

- 1 veal kidney 500 g

- Milk for inserting the kidney

- 1 onion 60 g, diced

- 1 clove of garlic, diced

- 2 tbsp olive oil

- 1 pinch brown sugar

- 150 ml white dry wine

- 50 g whipped cream

- 1 fresh bay leaf

- Salt

- Pepper from the mill

- 1 tbsp finely chopped tarragon

Directions:

1. Halve the veal's kidney longitudinally, parry, rinse well and cover for about 45 minutes with milk, then remove, pat dry, and cut into bite-sized pieces.
2. Heat-up oil in a pan, fry the kidney pieces quickly, remove them, and keep warm.
3. Sweat the onions plus garlic until translucent in the frying fat, sprinkle with the sugar, deglaze with wine, put in the bay leaf, and cook for 5 minutes.
4. Season with salt and pepper, remove the bay leaf and remove the sauce from the stove. Mix in the cream and half of the tarragon, add the juice and kidneys, and warm them up carefully.
5. Arrange the kidneys in a preheated bowl and serve the remaining tarragon sprinkled with it.

Nutrition:

Calories: 99

Protein: 15.76 g

Carbs: 0.85 g

Fats: 3.12 g

Zucchini Risotto with Kidneys

- ➢ Preparation time: 1 hour & 15 minutes
- ➢ Cooking time: 50 minutes
- ➢ Servings: 4
- ➢ Level of difficulty: Normal

Ingredients:

- 200 g pig kidney
- 1 shallot
- 2 tbsp oil
- 1 tbsp grass-fed butter
- 7 sage leaves
- 3 tbsp white dry wine
- salt
- pepper from the grinder

For the risotto:

- 700 ml vegetable broth (finished product)
- 1 onion
- 1 clove of garlic
- 80 g grass-fed butter
- 250 g pilaf rice
- 125 ml white wine
- salt
- pepper
- 1 zucchini
- 1 tbsp olive oil

Directions:

1. Brush the kidneys, rinse and cover with water for about 2 hours. For the risotto, bring the vegetable stock to the boil. Peel and dice the onion and garlic.

2. Heat 40 g butter in a saucepan. Steam the onion, garlic, and rice until translucent. Deglaze with white wine. Gradually pour in the broth while stirring so that the rice is always covered.

3. As soon as it has absorbed the liquid, pour in the broth again within 20-25 minutes. Stir in the remaining butter in pieces and season with salt and pepper.

4. Cover and let steep a little. Rinse, clean, and cut zucchini into pieces. Heat olive oil. Fry the zucchini in it for 3-4 minutes, season with salt and pepper, and mix with the risotto.

5. Pat the kidneys dry and cut into smaller pieces. Peel and dice shallot. Heat the oil and butter. Fry the kidneys in it for 12-15 minutes, adding the shallot cubes and the sage leaves.

6. Deglaze with wine, flavor with salt plus pepper. Serve the risotto with the kidneys.

Nutrition:

Calories 363

Protein 9.1 g

Carbs 71.2 g

Fat 4.1 g

Konjac Spaghetti with Broccoli

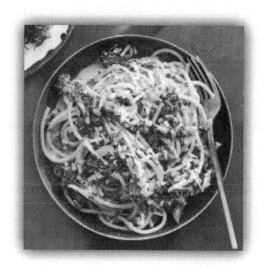

- ➢ Preparation time: 15 minutes
- ➢ Cooking time: 10 minutes
- ➢ Servings: 4
- ➢ Level of difficulty: Normal

Ingredients:

- 300 grams of Konjac spaghetti
- 400 gr of broccoli
- 3 tablespoons of extra virgin olive oil
- A pinch of whole sea salt
- 1 clove of garlic
- 4 anchovies in oil
- 10 gr of pine nuts
- 2 tablespoons of grated Parmesan cheese
- 2 tablespoons of grated pecorino Romano (an Italian cheese)
- 1 chili

Directions:

1. Clean the broccoli by dividing the florets, wash them, and put them in a pot containing 4 liters of lightly boiling salted water. After 6-7 minutes, they will be cooked, so drain them.

2. Brown the garlic clove with the oil and anchovies in a large pan. When it is golden, remove the garlic and add the chili, pine nuts, and broccoli. Allow to flavor by stirring.
3. Separately, cook the spaghetti in slightly salted boiling water. Drain them al dente and cook them in the broccoli pan.
4. Finally, season them with the grated parmesan and pecorino. Serve immediately.

Nutrition:

Calories 89

Protein 4.54 g

Carbs 8.1 g

Spaghetti with zucchini and champignons

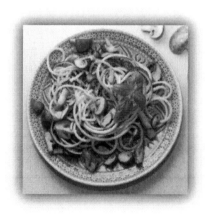

➢ Preparation time: 15 minutes
➢ Cooking time: 5 minutes
➢ Servings: 2
➢ Level of difficulty: Easy

Ingredients:

- 3 zucchinis
- 250 gr of champignons mushrooms
- ½ clove of minced garlic
- 2 tablespoons extra virgin olive oil

- Integral sea salt
- 80 gr of pecorino cheese
- A few basil leaves

Directions:

1. Wash the zucchini and cut into spaghetti
2. Wash the mushrooms and slice them
3. Heat a pan with a drizzle of oil and chopped garlic and sauté over high heat.
4. In a boiling pot of lightly salted water, plunge the zucchini and quickly scoop them out with an immersion colander or ladle. Place in a bowl and let cool.
5. Compose the dish with the zucchini spaghetti, mushrooms, extra virgin olive oil, pecorino cheese, and a few basil leaves to decorate.

Nutrition:

Calories 178

Protein 7.38 g

Carb 6.25 g

Asparagus in Salad with Poached Eggs

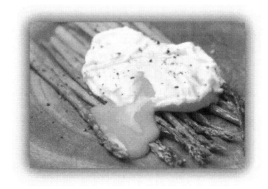

- ➤ Preparation time: 15 minutes
- ➤ Cooking time: 15 minutes
- ➤ Servings: 1
- ➤ Level of difficulty: Normal

Ingredients:

- 100 gr of asparagus already cleaned

- 1 fresh egg

- 1 tablespoon of apple vinegar

- A pinch of salt

For the dressing:

- 1 tablespoon of lemon juice

- 1 tablespoon of oil

- A modest bit of salt

- A grind of black pepper

Directions:

1. Carefully wash the asparagus in cold water, scrape the part of the stem with a small knife or a potato peeler and equalize them by breaking the final part with your hands, which will break by itself in the right place, to eliminate the hardest part.

2. Meanwhile, boil 3 liters of water in a pan large enough to hold the asparagus horizontally, throw in the asparagus and cook for 5-10 minutes.

3. Change the first cooking water with another slightly salted and boiling water. Cook for another 5 minutes. When they are cooked according to your taste, drain them gently, let them dry on a cloth, and finally arrange them on the plate.

4. Separately, cook the poached egg proceeding as follows: in a large saucepan, half full of boiling water, add a pot of salt and vinegar; lower the heat so that the water does not boil too strongly.

5. Then gently pour the egg that you have previously broken into a saucer. Using the skimmer, make sure that the egg white does not disperse.

6. Cook slowly for 2-3 minutes and then, again with a slotted spoon, remove the egg from the saucepan, pass it in ice water to stop cooking, drain and dry it gently with kitchen paper or a towel.

7. Separately, beat the sauce ingredients, arrange the egg on the asparagus plate and serve with the sauce separately.

Nutrition:

Calories 194

Protein 16.8

Carbs 5.8 g

Fat 11.7

Swordfish steak with lime and celery salad

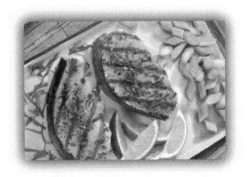

- ➤ Preparation: 15 minutes
- ➤ Cooking: 10 minutes
- ➤ Servings: 2
- ➤ Level of difficulty: easy

Ingredients:

- 2 slices of fresh swordfish
- 3 stalks of fresh celery
- ½ lime
- 1 tablespoon apple vinegar
- 2 tablespoons olive oil
- 1 pinch whole sea salt
- Red and black peppercorns
- A sprig of parsley

Directions:

1. Massage the swordfish slices with the salt, oil, and ground red and black pepper.
2. Heat a thick-bottomed skillet and cook the swordfish slices until they have reached the right browning, tinged with lime juice.
3. In the meantime, clean the celery stalks, slice diagonally and season with apple cider vinegar, salt and oil.

4. Pour the swordfish into a serving dish with the celery and add chopped parsley and a little more lime juice if desired.

Calories 195

Protein 19.5 g

Carbs 2.8 g

Fats 15.7 g

Tagliatelle with Courgettes and Pistachios

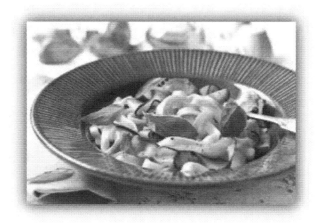

➤ Preparation time: 15 minutes
➤ Cooking time: 10 minutes
➤ Servings: 3
➤ Level of difficulty: Normal

Ingredients:

- 250 g of Konjac tagliatelle
- 500 g of already cleaned zucchini
- 50 g vacuum-packed pistachios, peeled and unsalted
- 40 g of grated Parmesan cheese
- 1/2 lemon
- 1 bay leaf
- A bunch of mints (for flavor and garnish only)

- Salt
- 4 tablespoons of extra virgin olive oil

Directions:

1. Slice the courgettes lengthwise and arrange them in strips on the oven plate. Salt lightly and sprinkle them with very little oil. Bake in the oven at 200 F within 8-10 minutes.
2. Coarsely chop the remaining zucchini and quickly brown it in a pan with a drizzle of oil and a tablespoon of water.
3. Add the pistachios and salt only if necessary.
4. Cook the Konjac tagliatelle in lightly salted boiling water for 10 minutes, by putting a lemon peel and bay leaf in the cooking water.
5. Drain it and pour into a large bowl. Add both the zucchini and pistachios to the bowl.
6. Season it by adding the parmesan, the mint leaves, the oil, and half a lemon juice. Serve.

Nutrition:

Calories 165

Protein 6.96 g

Carbs 22.74 g

Fat 6.46 g

Rice & Tuna Salad with Mediterranean Pesto

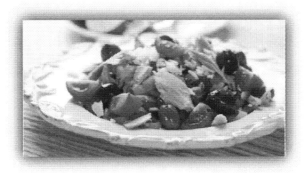

- ➤ Preparation time: 15 minutes
- ➤ Cooking time: 12 minutes
- ➤ Servings: 4
- ➤ Level of difficulty: Normal

Ingredients:

- 200 g of Basmati rice
- 150 g of tomatoes
- 80 g of courgettes
- 1 tablespoon of apple cider vinegar
- 2 drained tuna fillets
- A small pinch of salt for the rice cooking water
- A few drops of extra virgin olive oil to decorate

For the Mediterranean pesto:

- 40 g of pitted green olives
- 25 g of desalted capers
- 20 g of pine nuts
- 20 basil leaves
- 2 sprigs of fresh oregano
- A small fresh hot pepper, cleaned of seeds
- 1 clove of garlic
- 10 g of extra virgin olive oil

Directions:

1. Prepare the Mediterranean pesto by pounding the ingredients in a mortar or blending. Cook the low-protein rice, following the instructions on the package, and then shell it, allowing it to cool.
2. Clean the tomato and cut it into wedges.
3. Season the cooled rice with pesto, tomatoes, olives, tuna, and a tablespoon of apple cider vinegar.

Nutrition:

Calories 160

Protein 3.1 g

Carbs 18.8 g

Fat 8 g

Pizza Margherita gluten-free

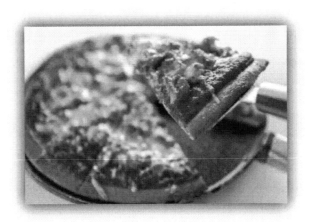

> ➤ Preparation time: 15 minutes
> ➤ Cooking time: 10 minutes
> ➤ Servings: 2
> ➤ Level of difficulty: Normal

Ingredients:

- 50 gr of coconut flour
- 20 gr of almond flour
- 3 eggs
- 25 gr of grated parmesan cheese
- 20 gr of ground flax seeds
- A pinch of oregano
- 125 gr of fresh tomato sauce
- A pinch of salt
- 80 gr of organic mozzarella
- Two tablespoons of EVO olive oil
- ½ teaspoon phosphate-free yeast

Directions:

1. Place the yeast, coconut, almond and flax seed flour, oil, eggs, salt, and Parmesan cheese in a blender. Let the mixture work for a few minutes, then pour it into a pizza pan. When the mixture is thick, it should be shaped with your hands on the pan directly.
2. Season with the tomato sauce, oregano, and a tablespoon of extra-virgin olive oil. Place in the oven at 350F for about 20 minutes, until the surface appears dark and crispy, then add the chopped mozzarella, put a few more minutes in the oven, bake and enjoy hot or warm.

Nutrition:

Calories 228

Protein 12.95 g

Carbs 16.05 g

Fat 9.77 g

Konjac "Alla Norma"

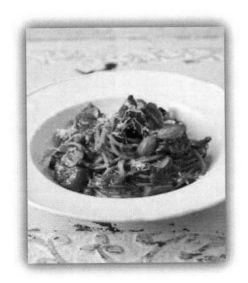

- ➤ Preparation time: 15 minutes
- ➤ Cooking time: 20 minutes
- ➤ Servings: 3
- ➤ Level of difficulty: Normal

Ingredients:

- 300 g of Konjac spaghetti
- 50 g of chopped onion
- 300 g of eggplant
- 400 g of tomato pulp
- 1 clove of garlic
- 4 tablespoons of extra virgin olive oil
- 40 g of pecorino Romano
- Chili pepper
- A pinch of salt

Directions:

1. Place Slice the eggplant into thin slices and pass them on a lightly greased plate or non-stick pan. Keep them aside.

2. Heat-up 3 tablespoons of olive oil in a large pan, add the clove of garlic and the finely sliced onion, brown, and add the tomato puree.

3. Put salt and chili, and cook for about 15 minutes. When cooked, add the eggplant slices and if you don't like it, remove the garlic clove. Meanwhile, cook your pasta in lightly salted water.

4. Once cooked, drain the pasta by collecting it from the pot with the special spaghetti collector tool and pass it, without draining it too much, into the pan with the sauce.

5. Sauté for a minute. Serve on hot plates and grate on each a few strands of pecorino Romano or salted ricotta cheese.

Nutrition:

Calories 88

Protein 2.5 g

Carbs 12.67 g

Fat 3.33 g

Whole grain penne with tuna

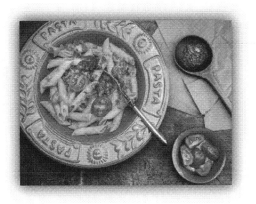

➤ Preparation time: 15 minutes
➤ Cooking time: 15 minutes
➤ Servings: 4

➤ Level of difficulty: Normal

Ingredients:

- 400 g of whole-grain penne
- 100 g of tuna in oil, already drained
- 1 clove of garlic
- 30 g of basil leaves
- 4 tablespoons of extra virgin olive oil
- 40 g of cherry tomatoes
- A pinch of salt

Directions:

1. Clean the basil and blend the leaves with two tablespoons of oil and a bit of salt.

2. Boil the pasta in salted water as stated in the package instructions. Taste it to check the cooking and keep it al dente to sauté it in a pan.

3. In the meantime, you have lightly fried the garlic with the remaining oil, add the well-drained tuna and the pureed basil.

4. When the pasta is cooked to the right point, drain it, keeping a little cooking water, and pass it a couple of minutes in the pan with the tuna and basil. Add the cherry tomatoes and serve.

Nutrition:

Calories 99

Protein 4.59 g

Carbs 15.52 g

Fat 2.12 g

Artichoke pilaf rice

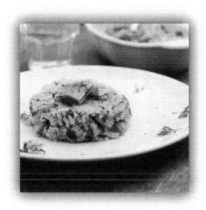

- ➢ Preparation time: 15 minutes
- ➢ Cooking time: 20 minutes
- ➢ Servings: 4
- ➢ Level of difficulty: Normal

Ingredients:

- 350 gr Pilaf rice
- 8 medium-sized artichokes
- 1 lemon
- about 25 oz of vegetable broth
- 2 shallots
- olive oil to taste
- salt

Directions:

1. Clean the artichokes by removing the hardest part of the stem, outer leaves and thorns.
2. Divide them into wedges and put them in a bowl with cold water acidulated with the juice of the squeezed lemon.
3. Chop the shallots and brown them for a few minutes in a little evo oil.
4. Add the artichokes and let them cook for 2/3 minutes.
5. Add a little hot water and cook the artichokes for 15 minutes until tender.
6. Now add the rice and let it toast for a couple of minutes.

7. Pour in the artichokes and broth, cover the pan and cook without stirring for 15 minutes: the rice will have absorbed all the liquid and will be cooked.

8. Prepare individual plates and pour the rice pilaf with artichokes using a pasta cup.

Calories: 184

Protein: 6 g

Carbs: 28 g

Fats: 10 g

Pizzoccheri light

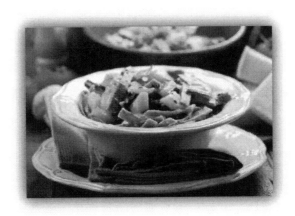

➢ Preparation time: 15 minutes
➢ Cooking time: 20 minutes
➢ Servings: 2
➢ Level of difficulty: Normal

Ingredients:

- 160 gr of pizzoccheri
- Sage
- 1 tbsp extra virgin olive oil raw
- 200 gr savoy cabbage
- 1 pinch of salt

- 1 pinch of mixed peppercorns to grind
- 2 tablespoons grated Parmesan cheese

Directions:

1. Select and wash the sage leaves.
2. Let them drain in a colander.
3. Dry them on a sheet of paper towels.
4. Pour the sage leaves into a small non-stick frying pan, with the flame off, and drizzle with a little oil so that they release their aroma.
5. Clean the Savoy cabbage, select the leaves and cut them into strips.
6. In a saucepan, bring plenty of salted water to the boil to cook first the Savoy cabbage and then the Savoy cabbage plus the pizzoccheri.
7. Pour in the Savoy cabbage and let it cook 10 minutes.
8. Add the pizzoccheri and let cook a couple of minutes less than the time indicated on the package.
9. Rinse pizzoccheri and Savoy cabbage under running water, drain thoroughly and pour into a bowl.
10. Add a pinch of salt, grind pepper and add a tablespoon of grated cheese, then mix.
11. Line a baking sheet with a sheet of crumpled baking paper.
12. Fill with pizzoccheri and Savoy cabbage, extra virgin olive oil and grated Parmesan cheese.
13. Heat oven briefly.
14. Bake at 350°F (180°C) for 15-20 minutes in a ventilated oven until the cheese is stringy and you get a crispy crust on the surface.

Calories: 454

Fat: 11.43 g

Carb.: 62 g

Protein: 19 g

Salad with Vinaigrette

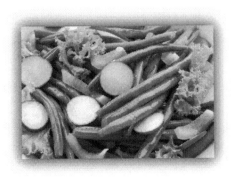

- ➢ Preparation Time: 25 minutes
- ➢ Cooking Time: 0 minutes
- ➢ Servings: 4
- ➢ Level of difficulty: Easy

Ingredients:

For the vinaigrette:

- ½ cup olive oil
- 4 tbsp balsamic vinegar
- 2 tbsp chopped fresh oregano
- pinch red pepper flakes
- ground black pepper

For the salad:

- 4 cups shredded green leaf lettuce
- 1 carrot, shredded
- ¾ cup green beans, cut into 1-inch pieces
- 3 large radishes, sliced thin
- ½ bell pepper, sliced

Directions:

1. For the vinaigrette, put the vinaigrette ingredients in a bowl and whisk.
2. In a bowl for the salad, toss together the carrot, lettuce, green beans, bell pepper and radishes. Put the vinaigrette on the vegetables, then toss to coat. Arrange the salad on plates and serve.

Nutrition:

Calories: 82

Carbs: 15 g

Protein:2 g

Fat:2 g

Cabbage and Cucumber Salad with Lemon Dressing

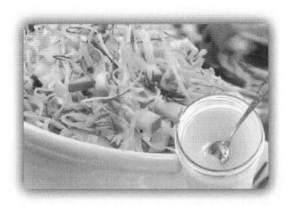

- ➤ Preparation Time: 10 minutes
- ➤ Cooking Time: 0 minutes
- ➤ Servings: 4
- ➤ Level of difficulty: Easy

Ingredients:

- ¼ cup of organic sugar-free cream
- 2 tbsp EVO oil
- ¼ cup freshly squeezed lemon juice
- 2 tbsp brown sugar
- 2 tbsp chopped fresh dill
- 2 tbsp finely chopped scallion, green part only
- ¼ tsp ground black pepper
- 1 English cucumber, sliced thin

- 2 cups shredded green cabbage

Directions:

1. Mix the lemon juice, cream, sugar, dill, scallion, and pepper until well blended in a small bowl.
2. Blend with a blender to make the sauce whipped and chop the flavors well.
3. Mix the cucumber and cabbage in a large bowl. Pour over the salsa at serving time

Nutrition:

Calories: 99

Carbs: 22g

Protein: 2g

Fat: 6g

Shrimp Salad with Mango and Lime

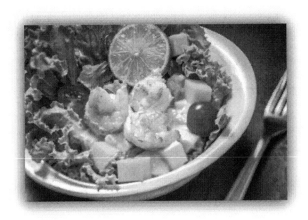

- ➢ Preparation Time: 15 minutes
- ➢ Cooking Time: 10 minutes
- ➢ Servings: 4
- ➢ Level of difficulty: Easy

Ingredients:

- 2 tbsp olive oil
- 6 oz large shrimp, peeled and deveined, tails left on
- 1 tsp minced garlic
- Curly lettuce leaves
- ½ cup chopped mango
- zest of 1 lime
- juice of 1 lime
- ground black pepper
- lime wedges for garnish

Directions:

1. Preheat a grill over medium heat. In a bowl, mix the olive oil, shrimp and garlic.
2. In a bowl, mix together the mango, slaw, lime zest and lime juice, and season the sauce lightly with pepper. Set aside.
3. Grill shrimp for 10 minutes, turning once or until shrimp are opaque and cooked through.
4. Season shrimp lightly with pepper. Place shrimp on salad with lime wedges on the side.

Nutrition:

Calories: 120

Carbs: 51g

Protein: 9g

Fat: 8g

Cabbage Stew

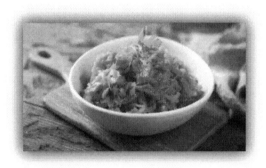

- ➢ Preparation time: 20 minutes
- ➢ Cooking time: 35 minutes
- ➢ Servings: 6
- ➢ Level of difficulty: Normal

Ingredients:

- 1 tsp grass-fed unsalted butter
- ½ large sweet onion
- 1 tsp minced garlic
- 6 cups shredded green cabbage
- 3 celery stalks, chopped with leafy tops
- 1 scallion, both green & white parts, chopped
- 2 tbsp chopped fresh parsley
- 2 tbsp freshly squeezed lemon juice
- 1 tbsp chopped fresh thyme
- 1 tsp chopped savory
- 1 tsp chopped fresh oregano
- water
- 1 cup carrots, sliced into pieces
- ground black pepper

Directions:

1. Melt the butter in a pot. Sauté the onion and garlic in the melted butter for 3 minutes, or until the vegetables are softened.

2. Add the celery, carrots, cabbage, scallion, parsley, lemon juice, thyme, savory, and oregano to the pot, add enough water to cover the vegetables by 4 inches.
3. Bring the soup to a boil. Reduce the heat to low and simmer the soup for 25 minutes or until the vegetables are tender. Put the green beans and simmer within 3 minutes—season with pepper.

Nutrition:

Calories:33

Carbs: 5g

Protein:1g

Fat:1g

Rice and Chicken Soup

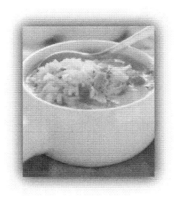

➢ Preparation time: 7 minutes
➢ Cooking time: 20 minutes
➢ Servings: 8
➢ Level of difficulty: Normal

Ingredients:

- 1 cup white onion, finely chopped
- 1 cup celery, diced
- 2 tbsp Extra virgin oil

- 1 cup baby carrot, chopped
- ½ tsp fresh ground black pepper
- ¾ cup white rice
- 1 bay leaf
- 4 fresh thyme sprigs
- 2 boneless skinless chicken breasts, cooked & cubed
- 10 cups no-salt-added chicken/vegetable broth
- 2 tbsp lime juice

Directions:

1. Sauté celery, carrot, and onion in olive oil in a large pot. Cook until softened. Cook rice. Add pepper, fresh thyme, bay leaf, rice, and stock. Bring to a boil.
2. Reduce heat and let simmer within 15 minutes. Add chicken and cook ten minutes more. Add lime juice. Remove bay leaf before serving.

Nutrition:

Calories 160

Protein 14g

Carbohydrates 19g

Fat 3g

Herbed Chicken

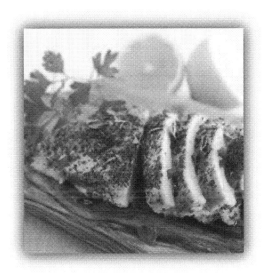

- ➢ Preparation Time: 20 minutes
- ➢ Cooking Time: 15 minutes
- ➢ Servings: 4
- ➢ Level of difficulty: Normal

Ingredients:

- 12 oz chicken breast, boneless & skinless, sliced into 8 strips
- 1 egg white
- 2 tbsp water, divided
- ½ cup breadcrumbs
- 3 tbsp ghee
- juice of 1 lemon
- zest of 1 lemon
- 1 tbsp freshly chopped basil
- 1 tsp freshly chopped thyme
- lemon slices, for garnish

Directions:

1. Put the chicken strips between 2 sheets of plastic wrap, then pound each flat with a rolling pin. Mix the egg and 1 tbsp water in a bowl.

2. Put the breadcrumbs in another bowl. Dip your chicken strips in the egg, then the breadcrumbs, and set the breaded strips aside on a plate.

3. Dissolve 2 tbsp of the ghee in your large skillet on medium heat. Cook the butter's strips for 3 minutes, turning once, or until they are golden and cooked through. Transfer the chicken to a plate.

4. Add the lemon zest, lemon juice, basil, thyme, and remaining 1 tbsp water to the skillet and stir until the mixture simmers.

5. Remove the sauce, then mix in the remaining tbsp ghee. Serve the chicken with the lemon sauce drizzled over the top and garnished with lemon slices.

Nutrition:

Calories:255

Carbs 83.6 g

Protein:20g

Fat:14g

Pesto Pork Chops

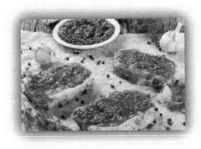

> ➢ Preparation Time: 20 minutes
> ➢ Cooking Time: 20 minutes
> ➢ Servings: 4
> ➢ Level of difficulty: Normal

Ingredients:

- 4 pork top-loin chops, 3-ounce boneless, fat trimmed

- 8 tsp herb pesto (basil, parsley, garlic, pine nuts, oil, salt, pepper)

- 2 tbsps olive oil

Directions:

1. Preheat the oven to 450F. Line a baking sheet with foil. Set aside. Rub 1 tsp of pesto evenly over both sides of each pork chop.
2. Lightly dredge each pork chop in the breadcrumbs. Heat the oil in a skillet. Brown the pork chops on each side for 5 minutes.
3. Put the pork chops on your prepared baking sheet. Bake for 10 minutes or until pork reaches 145F in the center.

Nutrition:

Calories:210

Carbs: 1g

Protein:24g

Fat:7g

Vegetable Curry

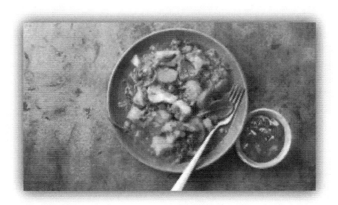

- ➤ Preparation Time: 15 minutes
- ➤ Cooking Time: 45 minutes
- ➤ Servings: 4
- ➤ Level of difficulty: Normal

Ingredients:

- 2 tsp olive oil
- ½ sweet onion, diced
- 2 tsp minced garlic
- 2 tsp grated fresh ginger
- ½ eggplant, peeled and diced
- 1 carrot, peeled and diced
- 1 red bell pepper, diced
- 1 tbsp hot curry powder
- 1 tsp ground cumin
- ½ tsp coriander
- pinch cayenne pepper
- 1 ½ cups vegetable stock
- 1 tbsp cornstarch
- ¼ cup of water

Directions:

1. Heat the oil in a stockpot. Sauté the ginger, garlic, and onion for 3 minutes or until they are softened.
2. Add the red pepper, carrots, eggplant, and often stir for 6 minutes. Stir in the cumin, curry powder, coriander, cayenne pepper, and vegetable stock.
3. Boil the curry, then lower the heat to low. Simmer the curry for 30 minutes or until the vegetables are tender.
4. Mix the cornstarch plus water in a bowl. Stir in the cornstarch mixture into the curry and simmer for 5 minutes or until the sauce has thickened.

Nutrition:

Calories:100

Carbs: 39g

Protein:1g

Fat:3g

Grilled Steak with Salsa

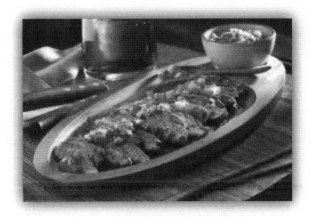

➢ Preparation Time: 20 minutes

➢ Cooking Time: 15 minutes

➢ Servings: 4

➢ Level of difficulty: Normal

Ingredients for the salsa:

- 1 cup chopped English cucumber
- ¼ cup boiled and diced red bell pepper
- 11 scallions, both green and white parts, chopped
- 2 tbsp chopped fresh cilantro
- juice of 1 lime

For the steak:

- 4 beef tenderloin steaks, 3-ounce, room temperature
- olive oil
- freshly ground black pepper

Directions:

1. For the salsa, mix the lime juice, cilantro, scallion, bell pepper, and cucumber in a bowl. Set aside.

2. For the steak, preheat a barbecue to medium heat. Massage the steaks all over with oil, then season with pepper.

3. Grill the steaks for about 5 minutes per side for medium-rare, or until the desired doneness. Serve the steaks topped with salsa.

Nutrition:

Calories:130

Carbs: 19g

Protein:19g

Fat:6g

Caraway Cabbage and Rice

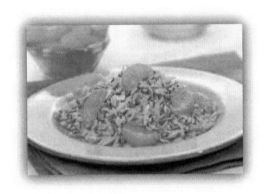

➢ Preparation Time: 5 minutes
➢ Cooking Time: 10 minutes
➢ Servings: 2
➢ Level of difficulty: Normal

Ingredients:

- 1 cup of whole grain rice, cooked
- ¼ cup mandarin oranges
- 1 tablespoon white onion, chopped
- 1 cup cabbage, shredded
- ½ teaspoon caraway seed
- 1 tablespoon Worcestershire sauce
- ¼ cup of water

Directions:

1. Take a frying pan, grease it with oil, place it over medium heat, add onion and cabbage and cook within 5 minutes until cabbage leaves wilted.

2. Stir in caraway seeds, Worcestershire sauce, and water, continue cooking for 3 minutes, add oranges and stir until rice until well combined. Serve straight away.

Nutrition:

Calories:142

Carbs: 18g

Potassium:194mg

Protein:3g

Fat:0g

Chicken and Sweet Potato Stir Fry

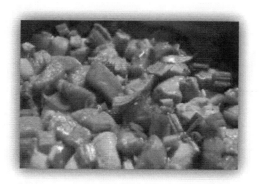

➤ Preparation Time: 15 minutes
➤ Cooking Time: 40 minutes
➤ Servings: 3
➤ Level of difficulty: Normal

Ingredients:

- ¼ teaspoon whole sea salt
- 1 garlic clove, minced
- 1 cup frozen peas
- 1 cup water
- 1 jalapeno pepper, chopped
- 1 medium onion, chopped
- 1 medium-sized red bell bell pepper, chopped
- 1 teaspoon cumin, ground
- 1/8 teaspoon black pepper
- 340 g boneless chicken
- 2 medium sweet potatoes
- 3 tablespoons olive oil
- 3 tbsp fresh cilantro, chopped

Directions:

1. In a small saucepan, place sweet potatoes with enough water to cover. Bring to a boil. Drain potatoes and discard water.
2. In a skillet, add the chicken and cook until golden brown. Transfer to a bowl. Using the same skillet, heat 2 tablespoons oil and sauté onions and jalapeno pepper for one minute.
3. Add the bell bell pepper, cumin and garlic: cook for three minutes until the vegetables have softened. Add the peas and chicken. Cook for two minutes before adding the sweet potato.
4. Stir cilantro and add salt and pepper to taste. Serve and enjoy.

Nutrition:

Calories: 375

Carbs: 39g

Protein: 28g

Fats: 18g

Chicken and Asparagus

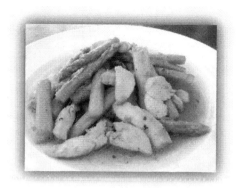

- ➢ Preparation Time: 5 minutes
- ➢ Cooking Time: 10 minutes
- ➢ Servings: 8
- ➢ Level of difficulty: Normal

Ingredients:

- 8 ounces skinless chicken breasts, cubed

- 16 ounces penne pasta, cooked

- 1pound asparagus spears, trimmed

- ½ teaspoon minced garlic

- ¼ teaspoon garlic powder

- ½ teaspoon ground black pepper

- 1 ½ teaspoons dried oregano

- 5 tablespoons olive oil

- ½ cup homemade chicken broth

Directions:

1. On medium-high heat, put a large skillet pan, add 3 tablespoons oil and when hot, add chicken cubes, stir in garlic powder and ¼ teaspoon black pepper and continue cooking for 5 minutes until cooked and browned.

2. When done, transfer chicken cubes to a plate lined with paper towels.

3. Then cook the chicken broth, add asparagus, season with oregano and remaining black pepper, and cook for 5 minutes until asparagus has steamed, covering the pan.

4. Let rest 10 minutes. Season with a little oil and serve.

Nutrition:

Calories:296

Carbs: 23g

Protein:18g

Fat:12g

Hawaiian Rice

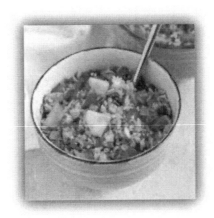

➢ Preparation Time: 5 minutes
➢ Cooking Time: 13 minutes
➢ Servings: 6
➢ Level of difficulty: Normal

Ingredients:

- ½ cup pineapple tidbits, unsweetened
- ½ cup red bell pepper, chopped
- ½ cup mushrooms, chopped
- 1 teaspoon ginger root, minced
- ½ cup bean sprouts
- ½ tablespoon soy sauce, reduced-sodium
- ¼ teaspoon salt
- 2 cups brown rice, cooked
- 1 green chili

Directions:

1. Take a frying pan, spray it with oil, place it over medium heat and when hot, put all the vegetables and cook within 5 minutes until sautéed.
2. Then stir in ginger and pineapple, drizzle with soy sauce, season with salt and cook for 3 minutes, or until hot. Stir in rice until well mixed, cook for 3 minutes until hot, and then serve.

Nutrition:

Calories:97

Carbs: 28g

Protein:2g

Fat:1g

Shrimp Fried Rice

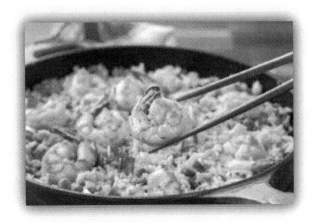

- ➢ Preparation Time: 5 minutes
- ➢ Cooking Time: 20 minutes
- ➢ Servings: 4
- ➢ Level of difficulty: Normal

Ingredients:

- 4 cups white rice, cooked
- ½ cup small frozen shrimp, cooked
- ¾ cup white onion, chopped
- 1 cup frozen peas and carrots
- 3 tablespoons scallions, chopped
- ½ teaspoon minced garlic
- 1 tablespoon ginger root, grated
- ¼ teaspoon salt
- ¾ teaspoon ground black pepper
- 5 tablespoons olive oil
- 4 eggs

Directions:

1. Put 1 tablespoon olive oil in a large skillet pan over medium-high heat, and when hot, add onion, season with ½ teaspoon black pepper, and cook for 2 minutes, or until onions are tender.

2. Stir in scallions, ginger, and garlic, cook for 1 minute, add shrimps, stir until mixed, cook for 2 minutes until hot, then stir in carrots and peas and cook for 2 minutes until hot.

3. When done, transfer shrimps and vegetable mixture to a bowl, cover with a lid, and set aside until required.

4. Move back the skillet pan over medium heat, add 2 tablespoons of oil, beat the eggs, pour it into the pan, cook for 3 minutes until eggs are scrambled to the desired level, and then transfer eggs to the bowl containing shrimps and vegetables.

5. Put the rest of the 1 tablespoon oil and when hot, add rice, stir until well coated, and cook for 2 minutes until hot.

6. Then season rice with salt and remaining black pepper, cook for 2 minutes, don't stir, then add eggs, shrimps, and vegetables, stir until mixed and cook for 3 minutes until hot. Serve straight away.

Nutrition:

Calories:421

Carbs: 55g

Protein:16g

Fat:16g

Meatloaf

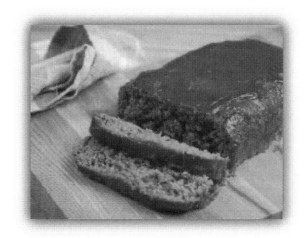

- ➤ Preparation Time: 10 minutes
- ➤ Cooking Time: 50 minutes
- ➤ Servings: 6
- ➤ Level of difficulty: Normal

Ingredients:

- 1-pound lean ground beef
- 2 tablespoons white onion, chopped
- ¼ teaspoon ground black pepper
- 1 tablespoon brown sugar
- 1 egg
- 1/3 cup tomato paste
- ½ teaspoon apple cider vinegar
- 2 tablespoons milk, low-fat
- 1 teaspoon water
- 25 gr unsalted breadcrumbs

Directions:

1. Switch on the oven, then set it to 350°F and let it preheat.
2. Take a large bowl, place beef, onion, and crackers in it, sprinkle with black pepper, pour in egg and milk, and stir until well combined.

3. Take a loaf pan, place beef mixture in it and bake for 40 minutes until cooked.

4. Meanwhile, prepare the sauce by placing tomate paste in a small bowl and whisk in vinegar, sugar, and water until combined.

5. When meatloaf has baked, cover its top with the prepared sauce and bake for 10 minutes until the top is glazed, and the internal temperature of meatloaf reaches 160°F.

6. When done, let meatloaf cool for 5 minutes, then take it out, slice it into six pieces, and serve.

Nutrition:

Calories 205

 Fat 9 g

Protein 17 g

Carbohydrates 14 g

Apple Spice Pork Chops

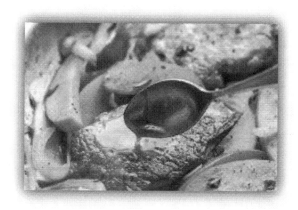

➢ Preparation Time: 10 minutes
➢ Cooking Time: 10 minutes
➢ Servings: 4
➢ Level of difficulty: Normal

Ingredients:

• 2 medium apples: peeled, cored, sliced

- 1-pound pork chops

- ¼ teaspoon marine salt

- ¼ cup brown sugar

- ¼ teaspoon ground nutmeg

- ¼ teaspoon ground black pepper

- ¼ teaspoon cinnamon

- 2 tablespoons unsalted grass-fed butter

Directions:

1. Switch on the broiler, let it preheat, then place pork chops in it and cook for 5 minutes per side until done.
2. Meanwhile, take a medium-sized skillet pan, place it over medium heat, add butter and when it melts, add apples, black pepper, salt, sugar, cinnamon, and nutmeg, stir well.
3. Cook within 8 minutes, or until apples are tender and the sauce has thickened to the desired level. When done, spoon the applesauce over pork chops and serve.

Nutrition:

Calories 306

Fat 16 g

Protein 22 g

Carbohydrates 21 g

Beef and turkey sausages with lemon sauce

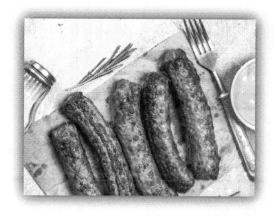

- ➢ Preparation: 15 minutes
- ➢ Cooking: 8 minutes
- ➢ Portions: 12
- ➢ Difficulty level: easy

Ingredients:

- 500 gr ground beef
- 250 g lean ground turkey meat
- ¼ teaspoon of nutmeg
- ½ teaspoon of black pepper
- ¼ teaspoon coriander
- 2 tablespoons maple syrup

Indications:

- Combine all ingredients in a bowl and mix. Cover and refrigerate for 3-4 hours. Take the mixture and form small cylinders with your hand (about 10-12).
- Lightly grease a medium greased skillet with oil and fry the patties over medium-high heat until browned for about 4-5 minutes on each side. Serve warm.

Lemon sauce ingredients:

- 6 tablespoons EVO oil
- 3 egg yolks
- 3 tablespoons lemon juice
- salt and pepper to taste

Preparation:

1. In a bowl, put the egg yolks, add the lemon juice and with the mixer create a cream.
2. Add the oil in a trickle, being careful not to make the sauce go crazy.
3. Add salt and pepper and continue to mix. Serve immediately.

Nutrition:

Calories: 53.85

Carbs: 2.42 g

Protein: 8.5 g

Fat: 0.9 g

Beef Burritos

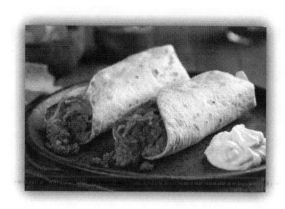

➤ Preparation Time: 10 minutes
➤ Cooking Time: 20 minutes
➤ Servings: 6
➤ Level of difficulty: Normal

Ingredients:

- ¼ cup white onion, chopped
- ¼ cup green bell pepper, chopped
- 1-pound ground beef
- ¼ cup tomato puree, low-sodium
- ¼ teaspoon ground black pepper
- ¼ teaspoon ground cumin
- 6 flour tortillas, burrito size
- sour cream for garnish

Directions:

1. Take a skillet pan, place it over medium heat, add beef, and cook for 5 to 8 minutes until browned. Drain the excess fat, then transfer beef to a plate lined with paper towels and serve.
2. Return pan over medium heat, grease it with oil and when hot, add pepper and onion, cook within 5 minutes, or soften.

3. Switch to low heat, return beef to the pan, season with black pepper and cumin, pour in tomato puree, stir until mixed and cook for 5 minutes until done.

4. Distribute beef batter evenly on top of the tortilla, roll them in burrito style by folding both ends, and then serve.

Nutrition:

Calories 265

Fat 9 g

Protein 15 g

Carbohydrates 31 g

DINNER RECIPES

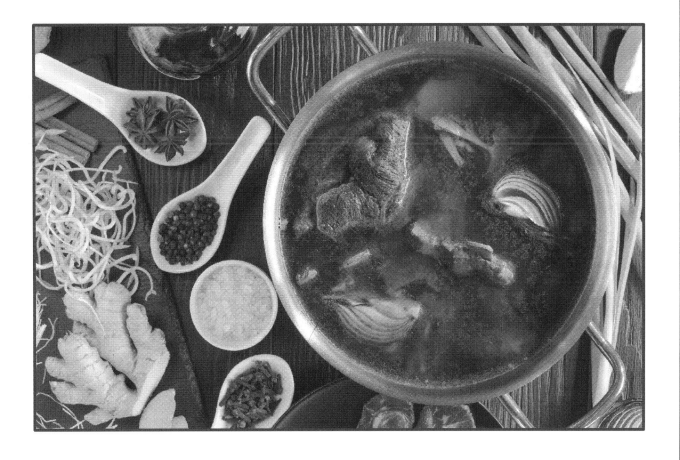

Broccoli and Beef Stir-Fry

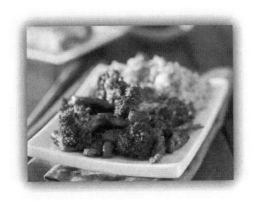

- ➤ Preparation Time: 5 minutes
- ➤ Cooking Time: 18 minutes
- ➤ Servings: 4
- ➤ Level of difficulty: Normal

Ingredients:

- 12 ounces frozen broccoli, thawed

- 8 oz sirloin beef, sliced into thin strips

- 1 medium Roma tomato, chopped

- 1 teaspoon minced garlic

- 1 tablespoon cornstarch

- 2 tablespoons soy sauce, reduced-sodium

- ¼ cup chicken broth, low-sodium

- 2 tablespoons peanut oil

- 2 cups cooked brown rice

Directions:

1. Take a frying pan, place it over medium heat, add oil and when hot, add garlic and cook for 1 minute until fragrant.

2. Add vegetable blend, cook for 5 minutes, then transfer vegetables to a plate and set aside until needed.

3. Add beef strips into the pan, and then cook for 7 minutes until cooked to the desired level.

4. Prepare the sauce by putting cornstarch in a bowl and then whisking in soy sauce and broth until well combined.

5. Returned vegetables to the pan, add tomatoes, drizzle with sauce, stir well until coated, and cook within 2 minutes until the sauce has thickened. Serve with brown rice.

Nutrition:

Calories 373

Fat 17 g

Protein 18 g

Carbohydrates 37 g

Fresh Cucumber Soup

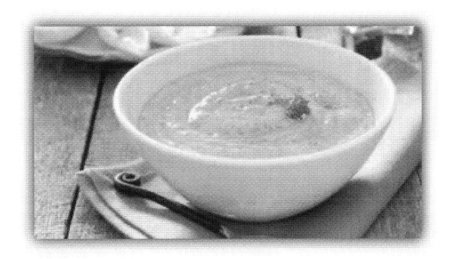

➤ Preparation Time: 2 hours 5 minutes
➤ Cooking time: 0 minutes
➤ Servings: 2
➤ Level of difficulty: Easy

Ingredients:

- 2 cucumbers, peeled & seeded
- 1/3 cup white onion, sliced
- 1 green onion, sliced
- 1/4 cup fresh mint, sliced
- 2 tbsp. Fresh lemon juice
- 2 tbsp. Fresh dill, sliced
- 2/3 cup water
- 1/3 cup sour cream
- 1/2 cup organic unsweetened whipping cream
- 1/2 tsp. Pepper
- 1/4 tsp. Salt

Directions:

1. Put all ingredients in a mixer and whisk until smooth. Cover and place in the refrigerator for at least 2 hours. Use fresh dill sprigs to garnish the soup. Serve and enjoy!

Nutrition:

Calories: 78

Protein: 2 g

Carbs: 17g

Fat: 11g

Potato, asparagus and strawberry salad

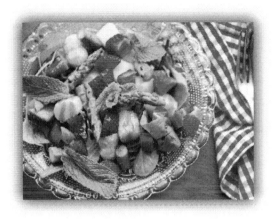

- ➤ Preparation Time: 15 minutes
- ➤ Cooking time: 30 minutes
- ➤ Servings: 4
- ➤ Level of difficulty: Easy
- ➤

Ingredients:

- 400 g of potatoes
- 500 g of green asparagus
- 1 cup sliced strawberries
- 1 handful of chervil, chopped
- 200 ml vegetable broth
- 2 tablespoons olive oil
- 4 tablespoons apple vinegar
- salt and pepper
- a few leaves of lettuce

Directions:

1. Wash the potatoes well and cook them for about 20 minutes in salted water.
2. Meanwhile, wash the asparagus, peel and cut off the hard ends of the bottom third. Cut sticks diagonally, about 2 inches long.

3. Cook for about 8 minutes in boiling salted water, then drain, rinse in cold water and drain.

4. Set aside about 4 stalks for garnish. Drain the potatoes at the end of cooking, rinse and peel them while they are still hot.

5. Slice the potatoes and add the asparagus stalks. Add the oil and apple cider vinegar to the salad, season with salt and pepper and season to taste.

6. Wash the lettuce leaves, shake them well and distribute them in the bowls. Arrange the asparagus tips and strawberries on top of the potato salad. Add some mint for garnish and serve.

Nutrition:

Calories 178

Protein 6 g

Fats 5 g

Carb. 25 g

Green Asparagus Soup

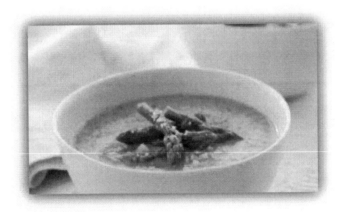

➤ Preparation time: 15 minutes
➤ Cooking time: 30 minutes
➤ Servings: 2
➤ Level of difficulty: Normal

Ingredients:

- 250 g green asparagus
- 1 shallot
- 10 g butter (1 tbsp)
- 400 ml classic vegetable broth
- 30 g parmesan (1 piece)
- ½ lemon
- 4 tbsp sour cream
- salt
- pepper
- 100 ml milk (1.5% fat)
- 3 drops truffle oil

Directions:

1. Wash and drain the asparagus and cut off any woody ends. Peel the asparagus in the lower third. Cut the sticks into pieces about 2 cm long. Peel and finely chop the shallot.

2. Heat the butter in a saucepan. Sauté the asparagus pieces and shallot in it over medium heat. Put in the vegetable stock and boil on low heat for about 15 minutes.

3. In the meantime, grate the parmesan cheese finely. Add the parmesan to the asparagus and finely puree everything with a hand blender.

4. Squeeze the lemon. Stir the soy cream into the soup, season with salt, pepper, and a little lemon juice.

5. Heat the milk, a pinch of salt, and truffle oil (to approx. 60 ° C), do not let it boil. Whip the milk until frothy using a hand blender.

6. Pour the soup into glasses or glass cups, distribute the milk foam on top. Serve immediately.

Nutrition:

Calories 197

Protein 10 g

Fat 14 g

Carb 6 g

Meatballs with Eggplant

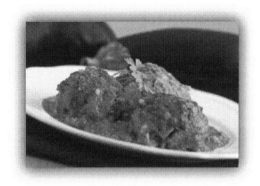

- ➤ Preparation Time: 15 minutes
- ➤ Cooking Time: 60 minutes
- ➤ Servings: 6
- ➤ Level of difficulty: Normal

Ingredients:

- 1-pound ground beef
- ½ cup green bell pepper, chopped
- 2 medium eggplants, peeled and diced
- ½ teaspoon minced garlic
- 1 cup stewed tomatoes
- ½ cup white onion, diced
- 1/3 cup olive oil
- 1 teaspoon lemon and pepper seasoning, salt-free
- 1 teaspoon turmeric

- 1 teaspoon Mrs. Dash seasoning blend
- 2 cups of water

Directions:

1. Take a large skillet pan, place it over medium heat, add oil in it, add garlic plus green bell pepper and cook within 4 minutes until sautéed.

2. Transfer green pepper mixture to a plate, set aside until needed, then eggplant pieces into the pan and cook within 4 minutes per side until browned, and when done, transfer eggplant to a plate and set aside until needed.

3. Take a medium bowl, place beef in it, add onion, season with all the spices, stir until well combined, then shape the batter into 30 small meatballs.

4. Place meatballs into the pan in a single layer and cook for 3 minutes, or until browned.

5. When done, place all the meatballs in the pan, add cooked bell pepper mixture in it along with eggplant, stir in water and tomatoes.

6. Simmer for 30 minutes at a low heat setting until thoroughly cooked. Serve straight away.

Nutrition:

Calories 265

Fat 18 g

Protein 17 g

Carbohydrates 12 g

Green pepper filet

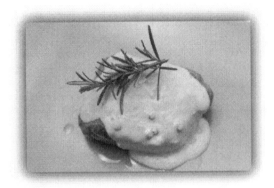

- ➤ Preparation Time: 10 minutes
- ➤ Cooking Time: 20 minutes
- ➤ Servings: 4
- ➤ Level of difficulty: Normal

Ingredients:

- • 1 kg beef fillet (4 fillets) at room temperature
- • 20 gr green peppercorns
- • 80 gr fresh liquid cream
- • 40 gr dijon mustard
- • 100 gr meat stock
- • 25 gr white wine
- • 20 gr ghee (clarified butter)
- • Salt to taste
- • Rice flour to taste

Directions:

1. 1 Pour the rice flour in a container and lay the fillets inside, taking care to flour only the top and bottom sides.
2. 2 Take a pan, add the ghee and let it melt on high heat.
3. 3 When the ghee is hot, place the fillets in the pan, sear them for a few moments over high heat, then lower the heat slightly and let them cook for 1-2 minutes without

touching them so that the first 6-7 mm of the fillet become golden brown. At this point raise the heat again and turn the fillets on the other side using a pair of tongs or two wooden spoons, without piercing the meat. Brown for a few more seconds, then cook for another 1-2 minutes over a lower heat. Finally, turn the fillets on their side and, turning up the heat again, roll them in the ghee so that the entire surface is sealed.

4. 4 At this point fade with the wine. Use a lighter and allow the alcohol to evaporate. Then lower the heat and add the green pepper, a pinch of salt, and mustard.

5. 5 Spread the seasoning all over the meat, then pour in 50 g of fresh cream and 50 g of stock and turn up the heat again.

6. 6 Move the pan to mix everything and continue cooking for a couple of minutes, continually basting the surface of the meat with the cream using a spoon. Then turn them over and do the same thing on the other side. For perfectly rare cooking, touch the surface of the fillet with a finger to make sure it is soft. If, on the other hand, you prefer the meat a little more cooked, extend the cooking time slightly by adding a little broth if necessary.

7. 7 Once the fillets are cooked, transfer them to serving plates and let them rest.

8. 8 In the meantime, take the pan with the cooking liquid, add the remaining 50 g of stock and 30 g of fresh cream, adjust the salt if necessary and let the sauce thicken over a high heat for 1-2 minutes, stirring the pan.

9. 9 At this point, take the plate with the fillet, sprinkle with a spoonful of cream and serve the fillet with green pepper immediately.

Nutrition:

Calories 441

Fats 26 g

Protein 48 g

Carb. 14 g

Barley and Beef Stew

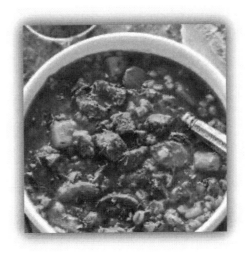

- ➢ Preparation Time: 10 minutes
- ➢ Cooking Time: 1 hour and 15 minutes
- ➢ Servings: 6
- ➢ Level of difficulty: Normal

Ingredients:

- 1-pound beef stew meat, 1 ½ inch, cubed
- 1 cup pearl barley, soaked for 1 hour
- ½ cup white onion, diced
- 2 medium carrots, peeled and sliced
- 1 large stalk of celery, diced
- 2 tablespoons rice flour
- ½ teaspoon minced garlic
- ¼ teaspoon ground black pepper
- ½ teaspoon salt
- 1 teaspoon onion herb seasoning
- 2 tablespoons olive oil

- 2 bay leaves

- 8 cups of water

Directions:

1. Place beef in a plastic bag, add rice flour and black pepper, seal the bag and shake well until well coated.
2. Take a large pot, place it over medium heat, add oil, and when hot, add coated beef and cook for 10 minutes until browned.
3. When done, transfer beef to a plate, add celery, onion, and garlic, cook for 2 minutes, pour in water, and bring the mixture to a boil.
4. Add beef into boiling mixture, then switch heat to medium level, season with salt, add bay leaf and barley to the pot, stir until mixed and cook for 1 hour until cooked through.
5. Half an hour from the end of cooking, add the barley to the pot and continue stirring occasionally so it doesn't stick.
6. Let the stew rest for 15 minutes and then serve.

Nutrition:

Calories 246

Fat 8 g

Protein 22 g

Carbohydrates 21 g

Chicken and Corn Soup

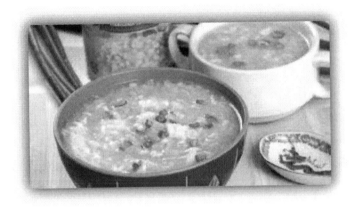

- ➤ Preparation Time: 15 minutes
- ➤ Cooking Time: 60 minutes
- ➤ Servings: 6
- ➤ Level of difficulty: Normal

Ingredients:

- 800 gr of chicken parts for broth
- 1 celery stalk
- 1 carrot
- ½ onion
- 1 bunch of parsley
- 1 tablespoon chopped chives
- 250 gr cooked organic corn
- ¼ teaspoon ground black pepper
- 1 liter of water

Directions:

1. In a large pot, pour the water, add the herbs (celery, onion, carrot, parsley) and the chicken pieces, cook for 40 minutes, and when ready, separate the chicken from the broth and set aside.
2. Remove the fat from the chicken broth by skimming it, let the chicken cool slightly and then cut it into pieces.
3. Take a large pot, place it over medium heat, pour in the broth, chicken pieces, add the corn, stir in the black pepper and parsley and simmer for 15-20 minutes.

4. When done, pour the soup into bowls and serve.
1. Take a thick bottom or cast-iron pot, put it over medium heat, add the butter and when it melts, add the onion and garlic and cook for 5 minutes, or until tender.
2. Then add the carrots, celery, stir in all the spices and herbs, continue cooking for 5 minutes.
3. Bring to low heat, incorporate the starch, continue cooking for 10 minutes, then pour in the wine and chicken stock and whisk until combined.
4. Add the chicken, gradually add the milk and continue to simmer for 15 minutes. When done, pour the rice into the soup and serve.

Nutrition:

Calories 222

Fat 6 g

Protein 25 g

Carbohydrates 17 g

Asparagus, Chicken and Wild Rice Soup

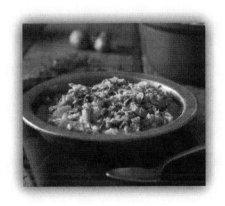

➢ Preparation Time: 10 minutes
➢ Cooking Time: 40 minutes
➢ Servings: 8
➢ Level of difficulty: Normal

Ingredients:

- 2 cups cooked and shredded chicken
- ¾ cup cooked wild rice
- ½ cup cornstarch
- 1 cup celery, diced
- 1 cup carrots, diced
- ½ cup white onion, diced
- 1 ½ teaspoons minced garlic
- ½ teaspoon salt
- ½ teaspoon dried thyme
- ½ teaspoon ground black pepper
- ½ teaspoon ground nutmeg
- 1 bay leaf
- ¼ cup of grass-fed butter
- ½ cup dry white wine
- 4 cups homemade chicken broth
- cups unsweetened almond milk

Directions:

1. Take a thick bottom or cast iron pot, put it over medium heat, add the butter and when it melts, add the onion and garlic and cook for 5 minutes, or until tender.
2. Then add the carrots, celery, stir in all the spices and herbs, continue cooking for 5 minutes.
3. Bring to low heat, incorporate the starch, continue cooking for 10 minutes, then pour in the wine and chicken stock and whisk until combined.
4. Add the chicken, gradually add the milk and continue to simmer for 15 minutes. When done, pour the rice into the soup and serve.

Nutrition:

Calories 185

Fat 11 g

Protein 21 g

Carbohydrates 28 g

Spicy Vegetable Stew

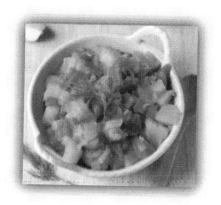

➢ Preparation Time: 20 minutes
➢ Cooking Time: 30 minutes
➢ Servings: 4
➢ Level of difficulty: Easy

Ingredients:

- 300 gr carrots
- 300 gr potatoes
- 300 gr zucchini
- 300 gr pumpkin
- 1 leek
- ½ teaspoon of mustard seeds
- 1 teaspoon cumin seeds
- 2 tbsp. sesame seeds
- 2 tbsp extra virgin olive oil
- 1 tbsp brown sugar
- 1 pinch of salt
- 2 tablespoons apple cider vinegar

Directions:

1. Wash the zucchini and cut into rounds, peel the potato, wash and dice it, peel the carrots and cut them into sticks. Peel and slice the leek, transfer to a colander, wash and drain well.

2. Peel the pumpkin and cut it into large cubes.

3. In a large skillet, pour in the oil, add the chiles and spices.

4. Cover the pan and sauté for a few minutes. Meanwhile, bring some salted water to a boil. Plunge the carrots and potatoes into the boiling water and cook for 10 minutes.

5. Moderate the heat of the pan with the spices and add the leek. Stir and let it brown for a few minutes. Now add the zucchini and squash, stir again and cook for a few minutes.

6. Salt the vegetables, then with a slotted spoon scoop out the potatoes and carrots and transfer them, little by little, to the pan, together with the other vegetables stirring gently.

7. Season with salt and pepper, add the brown sugar and cook over moderate heat for another 10 minutes. Stir occasionally. Finally season with the apple vinegar. Serve the stewed vegetables with spices piping hot.

Nutrition:

Calories 320

Fat 7 g

Protein 12 g

Carb. 54 g

Pumpkin Chili

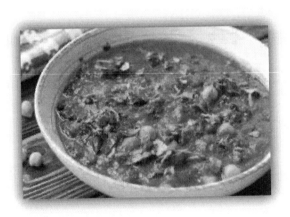

➤ Preparation Time: 10 minutes
➤ Cooking Time: 1 hour and 15 minutes
➤ Servings: 10

> Level of difficulty: Normal

Ingredients:

- 1 pound ground turkey
- 1 cup cooked kidney beans
- ½ cup white onion, chopped
- ½ cup green chilies, chopped
- ½ cup celery, chopped
- ½ cup carrot, sliced
- 1 ½ teaspoon minced garlic
- 1 tablespoon red chili powder
- 1 teaspoon dried oregano
- 2 teaspoons cumin
- 2 bay leaves
- 2 tablespoons olive oil
- 2 pound pumpkin puree
- 3 cups chicken homemade broth

Directions:

1. Take a large pot, place it over medium heat, add 1 tablespoon oil in it and when hot, add carrot, celery, onion, and garlic and cook for 5 minutes until tender and when done, transfer vegetables to a plate and set aside until needed.

2. Add remaining oil into the pot, add ground turkey, cook for 8 minutes, or wait until the meat is no longer pink.

3. Then stir in cooked vegetables and remaining ingredients, stir until mixed, switch to low heat, and cook for 1 hour, covering the pot. When cooked, remove bay leaf from the chili, then ladle it into bowls and serve.

Nutrition:

Calories 168

Fat 5 g

Protein 24 g

Carbohydrates 7 g

Cauliflower Manchurian

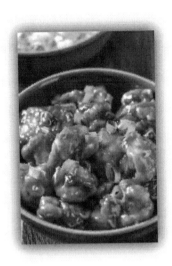

- ➢ Preparation Time: 10 minutes
- ➢ Cooking Time: 50 minutes
- ➢ Servings: 6
- ➢ Level of difficulty: Normal

Ingredients:

- 1 medium head of cauliflower, sliced into florets
- 1-inch piece of ginger root, grated
- ½ teaspoon minced garlic
- 1 teaspoon curry powder
- ½ teaspoon red chili powder
- ½ teaspoon cumin powder
- 2 tablespoons rice flour
- 1 teaspoon lemon juice
- 4 cups olive oil

Directions:

1. Take a heatproof bowl, place cauliflower florets in it, and microwave for 12 minutes at medium heat setting until soft. Then add flour, ginger, garlic, and all the spices, and then stir until well coated.

2. Take a deep pan, place it over medium-high heat, add oil, and when hot, add coated cauliflower florets in it and cook for 5 minutes, or until golden brown.

3. When cooked, transfer cauliflower florets to a plate lined with paper towels, cook remaining cauliflower in the same manner and then drizzle with lemon juice. Serve straight away.

Nutrition:

Calories 77

Fat 5 g

Protein 2 g

Carbohydrates 6 g

Eggplant Casserole

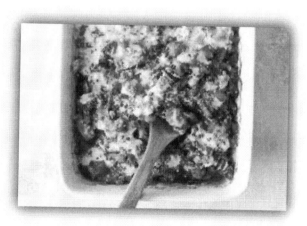

- ➢ Preparation Time: 10 minutes
- ➢ Cooking Time: 35 minutes
- ➢ Servings: 4
- ➢ Level of difficulty: Easy

Ingredients:

- 3 cups eggplant, diced
- 1/8 teaspoon salt
- ¼ teaspoon dried sage
- ½ teaspoon ground black pepper
- ½ cup breadcrumbs
- ½ cup liquid creamer, non-dairy
- 1 tablespoon margarine
- 3 eggs

Directions:

1. Switch on the oven, then set it to 350°F and let it preheat.

2. Meanwhile, place a large pot half full with water over medium heat, bring it to a boil, add eggplant pieces, cook for 5 to 8 minutes until boiling, and drain them.

3. Transfer eggplant pieces to a bowl, mash with a fork, whisk in salt, black pepper, sage, creamer, and eggs until mixed, and then spoon the mixture into a greased casserole dish.

4. Put your small frying pan on medium heat, add margarine and when it melts, add breadcrumbs and cook for 3 minutes until golden.

5. Spread breadcrumbs on top of eggplant mixture, then bake for 20 minutes until cooked through, and the top begins to look golden-brown. Serve straight away.

Nutrition:

Calories 186

Fat 9 g

Protein 7 g

Carbohydrates 19 g

Pineapple and Pepper Curry

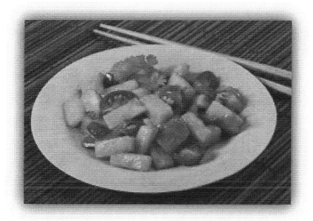

- ➢ Preparation Time: 5 minutes
- ➢ Cooking Time: 25 minutes
- ➢ Servings: 4
- ➢ Level of difficulty: Normal

Ingredients:

- 5 cherry tomatoes, halved
- 2 cups green bell pepper, chopped
- ½ cup pineapple pieces, with juice
- ½ cup red onion, chopped
- 1 tablespoon cilantro, chopped
- 1 tablespoon ginger root, grated
- 1 teaspoon curry powder
- ½ tablespoon lemon juice
- 2 tablespoons olive oil

Directions:

1. Take a medium-sized skillet pan and place it over medium heat, add oil, and when hot, add onion and ginger and cook for 7 minutes, or until softened.

2. Meanwhile, place the peppers in a heatproof bowl and microwave for 6 minutes on a high heat setting.

3. Add peppers into the onion mixture, stir well, switch to low heat, and cook for 10 minutes, stirring frequently.

4. Stir in pineapple pieces, simmer for 2 minutes, stir in cilantro and curry powder, stir again and simmer for 2 minutes until cooked.

5. When done, drizzle with lemon juice, garnish with cherry tomatoes, and then serve.

Nutrition:

Calories 107

Fat 7 g

Protein 1 g

Carbohydrates 10 g

Ratatouille

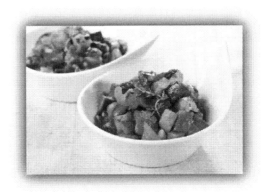

➢ Preparation Time: 10 minutes
➢ Cooking Time: 50 minutes
➢ Servings: 16
➢ Level of difficulty: Normal

Ingredients:

- 3 cups crookneck yellow squash, diced
- 2 cups white onion, diced
- 1 medium eggplant, diced

- 2 cups zucchini squash, diced
- 1 tablespoon sage leaves
- 2 medium carrots, peeled and diced
- 1 tablespoon rosemary leaves
- 1 tablespoon oregano leaves
- 1 tablespoon basil leaves
- 1 medium yellow bell pepper, diced
- 1 medium red bell pepper, diced
- 1 medium green bell pepper, diced
- 2 teaspoons minced garlic
- 2 tablespoons olive oil
- 1 cup tomatoes, diced
- 1 tablespoon ground black pepper
- 1 tablespoon thyme leaves
- 8 tablespoons parmesan cheese, grated

Directions:

1. Take a large skillet pan, place it over medium heat, add oil and when hot, add carrots, garlic, and all the herbs, season with black pepper and cook for 2 minutes.

2. Then add remaining vegetables, except for cherry tomatoes, stir and cook for 15 minutes, or until vegetables are tender-crisp.

3. Add tomatoes and cheese, stir until well mixed and simmer for 30 minutes until thoroughly cooked, covering the pan. Serve straight away.

Nutrition:

Calories 54

Fat 3 g

Protein 3 g

Carbohydrates 6 g

Brussels Sprouts with Pears

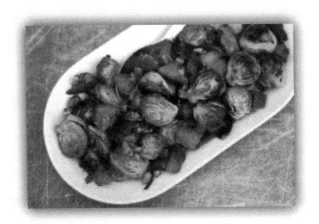

- ➢ Preparation Time: 10 minutes
- ➢ Cooking Time: 24 minutes
- ➢ Servings: 4
- ➢ Level of difficulty: Normal

Ingredients:

- 2 ½ cups Brussel sprouts, halved

- 2 medium pears, ½-inch cubed, peeled

- 2 teaspoons olive oil

- 1 teaspoon balsamic vinegar glaze

Directions:

1. Switch on the oven, then set it to 400°F, and let it preheat. Take a large bowl, add 1 teaspoon oil to it, then add sprouts and toss until well coated.

2. Take a 9 13 inches sheet pan, spread sprouts on one half in a single layer, and then bake for 12 minutes.

3. Add remaining oil in the bowl, add pear pieces to it, toss until well coated, and after 12 minutes, place pears on the empty side of the sheet pan.

4. Continue roasting for another 12 minutes, or until vegetables are tender. When done, drizzle glaze over the pears, toss them with sprouts, and then serve.

Nutrition:

Calories 110

Fat 3 g

Protein 2 g

Carbohydrates 19 g

Stuffed Zucchini

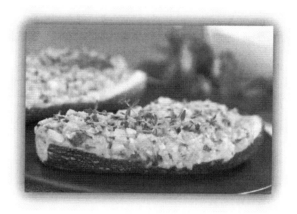

- ➢ Preparation Time: 10 minutes
- ➢ Cooking Time: 28 minutes
- ➢ Servings: 2
- ➢ Level of difficulty: Normal

Ingredients:

- • 4 slices of whole-grains bread, toasted

- • 2 medium zucchinis

- • ¼ teaspoon dried sage

- • 1 teaspoon onion powder

- • 1 teaspoon dill weed

- • 1 teaspoon lemon and pepper seasoning, salt-free

- 1 teaspoon Dash seasoning blend

Directions:

1. Prepare the zucchini by cutting each into half, lengthwise, and then scooping out the seeds to create a trench.
2. Take a medium-sized pot half full with water, place it over medium heat, bring it to a boil, add zucchini in it and boil for 3 to 5 minutes.
3. Meanwhile, toast the bread slices, transfer them to a food processor, and pulse until the mixture resembles crumbs.
4. Transfer breadcrumbs in a bowl, add sage, onion powder, dill, lemon and pepper, and Dash seasoning, and stir until mixed.
5. Drain the zucchini, pour ½ cup of the cooking liquid into the breadcrumb's mixture and blend with a fork until combined.
6. Take an 8-by-8 inches baking dish, place zucchini halves in it, peel side down, spoon breadcrumbs mixture into the zucchini, and then bake for 20 minutes until cooked. Serve straight away.

Nutrition:

Calories 82

Fat 1 g

Protein 3 g

Carbohydrates 15 g

Thai Red Curry Vegetables and Rice

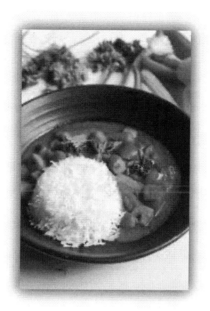

- ➢ Preparation Time: 10 minutes
- ➢ Cooking Time: 50 minutes
- ➢ Servings: 4
- ➢ Level of difficulty: Normal

Ingredients:

- • 2 cups cooked white rice
- • 1 cup green beans, diced
- • 1 small shallot, peeled and minced
- • 2 cups cauliflower florets
- • 2 medium carrots, sliced
- • 1 lime, cut into wedges
- • 1 lime leaf, dried
- • 2 tablespoons Thai red curry paste
- • 1 tablespoon canola oil
- • 14 ounces vegetable homemade broth
- • 8 ounces coconut milk, unsweetened

Directions:

1. Take a large pot, place it over low heat, add oil, and when hot, add shallots and cook within 8 minutes, or until tender.
2. Then stir in red curry paste, continue cooking for 1 minute until fragrant, add a lime leaf, pour in broth and milk, stir until mixed, and bring the mixture to a boil.
3. Add all the vegetables, stir until mixed, simmer for 12 minutes until vegetables are fork-tender and when done, remove the lime leaf.
4. Distribute rice between bowls, top with cooked vegetables and the sauce, and serve.

Nutrition:

Calories 210

Fat 17 g

Protein 8 g

Carbohydrates 26 g

Vegetable Paella

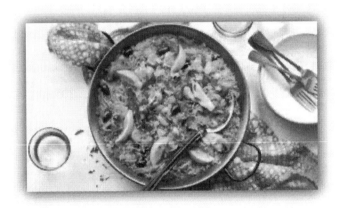

- ➢ Preparation Time: 5 minutes
- ➢ Cooking Time: 20 minutes
- ➢ Servings: 8
- ➢ Level of difficulty: Normal

Ingredients:

- 4 cups cooked thai rice
- 2 cups asparagus
- ½ cup white onion, chopped
- 1 cup green bell pepper, chopped
- 3 cups broccoli florets
- 1 ½ cup zucchini, chopped
- ½ teaspoon salt
- 1 tablespoon olive oil
- ½ teaspoon saffron

Directions:

1. Take a large pot, add broccoli and asparagus, pour in water to cover the vegetables, boil them for 4 minutes until tender-crisp, and drain them.

2. Take a large skillet pan, place it over medium heat, add oil, and when hot, add boiled vegetables along with onion, zucchini, and bell pepper and cook for 5 minutes until tender-crisp.

3. Then add remaining ingredients, stir until mixed and continue cooking for 5 minutes until hot. Serve straight away.

Nutrition:

Calories 146

Fat 2 g

Protein 5 g

Carbohydrates 26 g

Eggplant and Red Pepper Soup

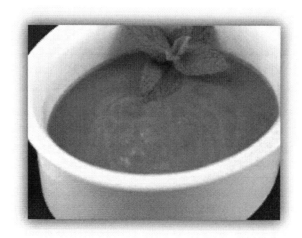

- ➢ Preparation Time: 20 minutes
- ➢ Cooking Time: 40 minutes
- ➢ Servings: 6
- ➢ Level of difficulty: Normal

Ingredients:

- 1 small sweet onion, cut into quarters
- 2 small red bell peppers, halved
- 2 cups cubed eggplant
- 2 cloves garlic, crushed
- 1 tbsp olive oil
- 1 cup chicken stock
- Water
- ¼ cup chopped fresh basil
- Ground black pepper

Directions:

1. Preheat the oven to 350F. Put the onions, red peppers, eggplant, and garlic in a baking dish. Drizzle the vegetables with the olive oil.

2. Roast the vegetables within 30 minutes or until they are slightly charred and soft. Cool the vegetables slightly and remove the skin from the peppers.

3. Puree the vegetables with a hand mixer (with the chicken stock). Transfer the soup to a medium pot and add enough water to reach the desired thickness.

4. Heat the soup to a simmer and add the basil. Season with pepper and serve.

Nutrition:

Calories: 61

Fat: 2g

Carb: 9g

Protein: 2g

Seafood Casserole

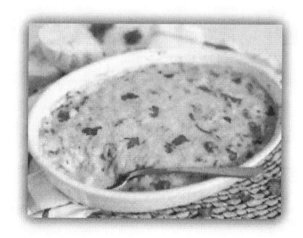

➢ Preparation Time: 20 minutes
➢ Cooking Time: 45 minutes
➢ Servings: 6
➢ Level of difficulty: Normal

Ingredients:

- 2 cups of eggplant peeled and diced into 1-inch pieces
- Butter, for greasing the baking dish
- 1 tbsp olive oil

- ½ sweet onion, chopped
- 1 tsp minced garlic
- 1 celery stalk, chopped
- ½ red bell pepper, boiled and chopped
- 3 tbsp freshly squeezed lemon juice
- 1 tsp hot sauce
- ¼ tsp Creole seasoning mix
- ½ cup white rice, uncooked
- 1 large egg
- 4 ounces cooked shrimp
- 6 ounces Queen crab meat

Directions:

1. Preheat the oven to 350F. Boil the eggplant in a saucepan for 5 minutes. Drain and set aside.

2. Grease a 9-by-13-inch baking dish with butter and set aside—heat-up olive oil in a large skillet over medium heat.

3. Sauté the garlic, onion, celery, and bell pepper for 4 minutes or until tender. Add the sautéed vegetables to the eggplant, along with the lemon juice, hot sauce, seasoning, rice, and egg. Stir to combine. Fold in the shrimp and crab meat.

4. Spoon the casserole mixture into the casserole dish, patting down the top. Bake for 25 to 30 minutes or until casserole is heated through and rice is tender. Serve warm.

Nutrition:

Calories: 61

Fat: 2g

Carb: 9g

Protein: 2g

Ground Beef and Rice Soup

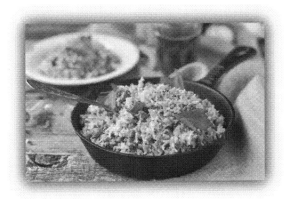

- ➤ Preparation Time: 15 minutes
- ➤ Cooking Time: 40 minutes
- ➤ Servings: 6
- ➤ Level of difficulty: Normal

Ingredients:

- ½ pound extra-lean ground beef
- ½ small sweet onion, chopped
- 1 tsp minced garlic
- 2 cups of water
- 1 cup homemade beef broth
- ½ cup long-grain white rice, uncooked
- 1 celery stalk, chopped
- ½ cup Fresh green beans, cut into – 1-inch pieces
- 1 tsp chopped fresh thyme
- Ground black pepper

Directions:

1. Sauté the ground beef in a saucepan for 6 minutes or until the beef is completely browned. Drain off the extra fat, then put the onion and garlic in the saucepan. Sauté the vegetables for about 3 minutes, or until they are softened.

2. Add the celery, rice, beef broth, and water. Boil the soup, reduce the heat to low, and simmer for 30 minutes or until the rice is tender.

3. Add the green beans and thyme and simmer for3 minutes. Remove the soup from the heat and season with pepper.

Nutrition:

Calories: 51

Fat: 2g

Carb: 9g

Protein: 2g

Couscous Burgers

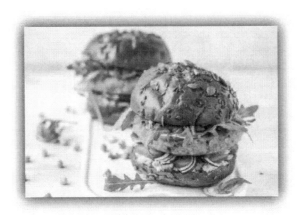

- ➢ Preparation Time: 20 minutes
- ➢ Cooking Time: 10 minutes
- ➢ Servings: 4
- ➢ Level of difficulty: Normal

Ingredients:

- ½ cup canned chickpeas, rinsed and drained
- 2 lightly beaten eggs
- 4 hamburger buns, whole grain
- 2 cups arugula leaves
- 2 tbsp chopped fresh cilantro
- Chopped fresh parsley

- 1 tbsp. lemon juice
- 1 tsp lemon zest
- 1 tsp minced garlic
- 1 ½ cups cooked couscous
- 2 tbsp olive oil

Directions:

1. Put the cilantro, chickpeas, parsley, lemon juice, lemon zest, and garlic in a food processor and pulse until a paste form.

2. Transfer the chickpea batter to a bowl and add the eggs and couscous. Mix well. Chill the batter in the refrigerator within 1 hour.

3. Form the couscous mixture into 4 patties—heat olive oil in a skillet. Put the patties in the skillet, two at a time, gently pressing them down with a spatula.

4. Cook within 5 minutes or until golden and flip the patties over. Cook the other side within 5 minutes and transfer the cooked burgers to a plate covered with a paper towel. Repeat with the remaining 2 burgers. Open the two buns in half, spread with a teaspoon of mustard and place the arugula leaves, sliced onion and burgers.

Nutrition:

Calories: 61

Fat: 2g

Carb: 9g

Protein: 2g

Baked Flounder

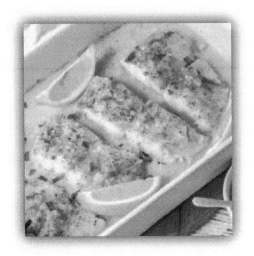

> ➢ Preparation Time: 20 minutes
> ➢ Cooking Time: 5 minutes
> ➢ Servings: 4
> ➢ Level of difficulty: Normal

Ingredients:

- 1 egg yolk
- 4 tbsp olive oil
- 1 tbsp apple vinegar
- 1 pinch of whole sea salt
- juice and zest of 1 lemon
- ½ cup chopped fresh cilantro
- 4 flounder fillets
- ground black pepper

Directions:

1. Preheat the oven to 400F. In a bowl, stir together the cilantro, lime juice, lime zest, and apple vinegar, salt, olive oil and the egg yolk.

2. Place a flounder fillet in a baking dish, then top the fillets evenly with the prepared mixture. Season the flounder with pepper and place an aluminum foil on top.

3. Bake the fish within 5 to 6 minutes. Leave it rest a couple of minutes, then serve.

Nutrition:

Calories: 51

Fat: 2g

Carb: 9g

Protein: 2g

Persian Chicken

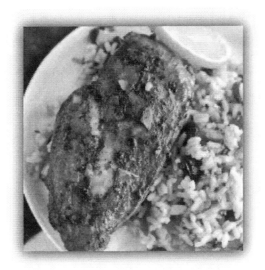

- ➢ Preparation Time: 10 minutes
- ➢ Cooking Time: 20 minutes
- ➢ Servings: 5
- ➢ Level of difficulty: Normal

Ingredients:

- ½ sweet onion, chopped
- ¼ cup lemon juice
- 1 tbsp dried oregano
- 1 tsp minced garlic
- 1 tsp sweet paprika
- ½ tsp ground cumin

- ½ cup olive oil
- 5 boneless, skinless chicken thighs

Directions:

1. Put the cumin, paprika, garlic, oregano, lemon juice, and onion in a food processor and pulse to mix the ingredients.

2. Keep the motor running and put the olive oil until the batter is smooth. Put the chicken thighs in a large sealable freezer bag and pour the marinade into the bag.

3. Seal it, then put it in the fridge, turning the bag twice, within 2 hours. Remove the thighs, then discard the extra marinade.

4. Warm barbecue grill to medium. Grill the chicken within 20 minutes, turning once, until it reaches 165F. Serve with rice on side, if desired.

Nutrition:

Calories: 321

Fat: 21g

Carb: 3g

Protein: 22g

Souvlaki Pork Skewers

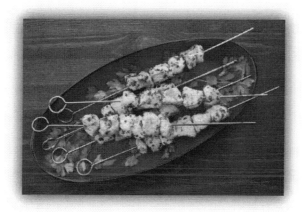

- ➤ Preparation Time: 20 minutes
- ➤ Cooking Time: 12 minutes
- ➤ Servings: 8
- ➤ Level of difficulty: Normal

Ingredients:

- 3 tbsp olive oil
- 2 tbsp lemon juice
- 1 tsp minced garlic
- 1 tbsp chopped fresh oregano
- ¼ tsp ground black pepper
- Pork leg – 1 pound, cut into 2-inch cubes

Directions:

1. In a bowl, stir together the lemon juice, olive oil, garlic, oregano, and pepper. Add the pork cubes and toss to coat.

2. Place the bowl in the refrigerator, covered, for 2 hours to marinate. Thread the pork chunks onto 8 wooden skewers that have been soaked in water.

3. Preheat the barbecue to medium-high heat. Grill the pork skewers for about 12 minutes, turning once, until just cooked through but still juicy.

Nutrition:

Calories: 61

Fat: 2g

Carb: 9g

Protein: 2g

Chicken Stew

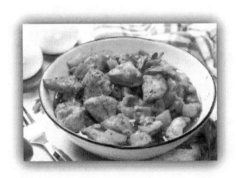

- ➢ Preparation Time: 20 minutes
- ➢ Cooking Time: 50 minutes
- ➢ Servings: 6
- ➢ Level of difficulty: Normal

Ingredients:

- 1 tbsp olive oil
- 1-pound boneless, skinless chicken thighs, cut into 1-inch cubes
- ½ sweet onion, chopped
- 1 tbsp minced garlic
- 2 cups homemade chicken stock
- 1 cup plus 2 tbsp water
- 1 carrot, sliced
- 2 stalks celery, sliced

- 1 turnip, sliced thin

- 1 tbsp chopped fresh thyme

- 1 tsp chopped fresh rosemary

- 2 tsp of cornstarch

- ground black pepper to taste

Directions:

1. Put your large saucepan on medium heat, then put the olive oil. Sauté the chicken for 6 minutes or until it is lightly browned, stirring often.

2. Put the onion plus garlic, and sauté for 3 minutes. Add 1-cup water, chicken stock, carrot, celery, and turnip, and bring the stew to a boil.

3. Adjust the heat to low, then simmer within 30 minutes or until the chicken is cooked through and tender. Add the thyme and rosemary and simmer for 3 minutes more.

4. In a small bowl, stir together the 2 tbsp of water and the cornstarch; add the mixture to the stew.

5. Stir to incorporate the cornstarch mixture and cook for 3 to 4 minutes or until the stew thickens. Remove, then flavor it with pepper. Serve.

Nutrition:

Calories: 141

Fat: 8g

Carb: 5g

Protein: 9g

Beef Chili

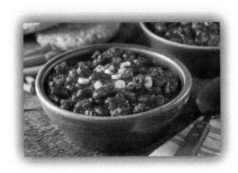

- ➢ Preparation Time: 10 minutes
- ➢ Cooking Time: 30 minutes
- ➢ Servings: 2
- ➢ Level of difficulty: Normal

Ingredients:

- 1 onion, diced
- 1 red bell pepper, diced
- 2 cloves garlic, minced
- 6 oz lean ground beef
- 1 tsp chili powder
- 1 tsp oregano
- 2 tbsp extra virgin olive oil
- 1 cup of water
- 1 cup of brown rice
- 1 tbsp Fresh cilantro to serve

Directions:

1. Soak vegetables in warm water. Boil a pan of water, then add rice for 20 minutes. Meanwhile, add the oil to a pan and heat on medium-high heat.
2. Add the pepper, onions, and garlic and sauté for 5 minutes until soft. Remove and set aside. Put the beef in the pan and stir until browned.
3. Add the vegetables back into the pan and stir. Now add the chili powder and herbs and the water, cover, and turn the heat down a little to simmer for 15 minutes.
4. Meanwhile, strain the water from the rice and the lid and steam while the chili is cooking. Serve hot with the fresh cilantro sprinkled over the top.

Nutrition:

Calories: 61

Fat: 2g

Carb: 9g

Protein: 2g

Shrimp Paella with Brown Rice

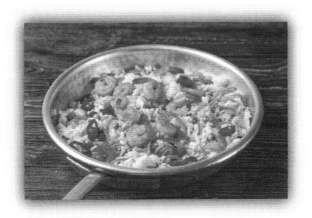

➤ Preparation Time: 5 minutes
➤ Cooking Time: 10 minutes
➤ Servings: 2
➤ Level of difficulty: Normal

Ingredients:

- 1 cup cooked brown rice
- 1 chopped red onion
- 1 tsp. paprika
- 1 chopped garlic clove
- 1 tbsp. olive oil
- 6 oz. frozen cooked shrimp
- 1 deseeded and sliced chili pepper

- 1 tbsp. oregano

Directions:

1. Heat-up olive oil in a large pan on medium-high heat. Add the onion and garlic and sauté for 2-3 minutes until soft.
2. Now add the shrimp and sauté for a further 5 minutes or until hot through. Now add the herbs, spices, chili, and rice with 1/2 cup boiling water.
3. Stir until everything is warm and the water has been absorbed. Plate up and serve.

Nutrition:

Calories 221

Protein 17g

Carbs 31g

Fat 8g

Salmon & Pesto Salad

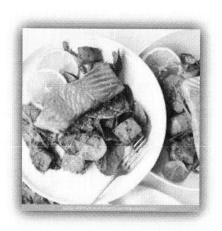

- ➢ Preparation Time: 5 minutes
- ➢ Cooking Time: 15 minutes
- ➢ Servings: 2
- ➢ Level of difficulty: Normal

Ingredients:

For the pesto:

- 1 minced garlic clove
- ½ cup fresh arugula
- ¼ cup extra virgin olive oil
- ½ cup fresh basil
- 1 tsp. black pepper

For the salmon:

- 4 oz. skinless salmon fillet
- 1 tbsp. coconut oil

For the salad:

- ½ juiced lemon
- 2 sliced radishes
- ½ cup iceberg lettuce
- 1 tsp. black pepper

Directions:

1. Prepare the pesto by blending all fixings in a food processor or grinding with a pestle and mortar. Set aside.
2. Add a skillet to the stove on medium-high heat and melt the coconut oil. Add the salmon to the pan.   Cook for 7-8 minutes and turn over.
3. Cook within 3-4 minutes or until cooked through. Remove fillets from the skillet and allow to rest. Mix the lettuce and the radishes and squeeze over the juice of ½ lemon.
4. Flake the salmon using a fork, then mix through the salad. Toss to coat, then sprinkle with a little black pepper to serve.

Nutrition:

Calories 221

Protein 13 g

Carbs 1 g

Fat 34 g

Baked Fennel & Garlic Sea Bass

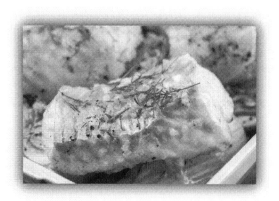

- ➤ Preparation Time: 5 minutes
- ➤ Cooking Time: 15 minutes
- ➤ Servings: 2
- ➤ Level of difficulty: Normal

Ingredients:

- 7 oz. sea bass fillets
- 1 lemon
- ½ sliced fennel bulb
- 1 tsp. black pepper
- 2 garlic cloves

Directions:

1. Preheat the oven to 375°F. Sprinkle black pepper over the Sea Bass. Slice the fennel bulb and garlic cloves.

2. Add 1 salmon fillet and half the fennel and garlic to one sheet of baking paper or tin foil. Squeeze in 1/2 lemon juices.

3. Repeat for the other fillet. Fold and add to the oven for 12-15 minutes or until fish is thoroughly cooked through.

4. Meanwhile, add boiling water to your couscous, cover, and allow to steam. Serve with your choice of rice or salad.

Nutrition:

Calories 221

Protein 14 g

Carbs 3 g

Fat 2 g

Lemon, Garlic & Cilantro Tuna and Rice

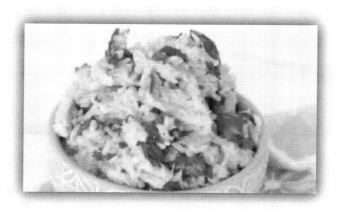

➤ Preparation Time: 5 minutes
➤ Cooking Time: 15 minutes
➤ Servings: 2
➤ Level of difficulty: Easy

Ingredients:

- 100 gr sea bass fillet
- 1/2 cup basmati rice
- ½ cup arugula
- 1 tablespoon extra-virgin olive oil
- 1 teaspoon black pepper
- ¼ finely chopped onion

- 1 lemon, squeezed
- tablespoons chopped fresh coriander

Directions:

1. Cook rice in boiling salted water 10 minutes. Drain and cool under running water. Pour the olive oil into a skillet, with the finely chopped onion, and sauté lightly.
2. Pour in the sea bass fillets and blanch for 5 minutes, drizzling with lemon juice.
3. Add the cooked rice and continue to stir-fry for a further 4 minutes or until the rice is hot.
4. At this point, add the arugula, pepper and coriander and turn off the heat. Cover and leave to rest for a few minutes. Serve warm.

Nutrition:

Calories 221

Protein 11 g

Carb. 26 g

Fats 7 g

Cod & Green Bean Risotto

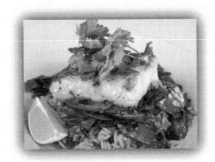

- ➤ Preparation Time: 4 minutes
- ➤ Cooking Time: 45 minutes
- ➤ Servings: 2

➤ Level of difficulty: Normal

Ingredients:

- 180 gr of cod fillet
- 1 finely chopped white onion
- 1 cup of mixed wild rice
- -2 lemon wedges
- 1 cup boiling water
- 1 cup vegetable broth
- ¼ teaspoon black pepper
- 3 tablespoons extra virgin olive oil
- 1 cup green beans

Directions:

1. Clean the green beans and cook them in water for 15 minutes. Drain and roast them in a small skillet freshly greased with oil for 5 minutes.
2. Heat the olive oil in a large skillet over medium heat. Sauté the chopped onion for 5 minutes until soft before adding the rice and stirring for 1-2 minutes.
3. Combine the broth with the boiling water. Add half of the liquid to the pan and stir slowly. Slowly add the rest of the liquid while stirring continuously for 30 minutes.
4. Stir the green beans into the risotto.
5. Heat a grill and cook the cod fillets in it lightly marinated in oil, pepper and lemon.
6. Place the fish on top of the rice, sprinkle with freshly ground pepper and a squeeze of fresh lemon. Garnish with the lemon wedges and a bunch of parsley.

Nutrition:

Calories 221

Protein 12 g

Carb. 29 g

Fats 8 g

Sardine Fish Cakes

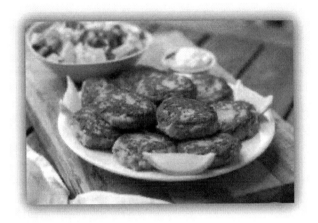

> ➤ Preparation Time: 10 minutes
> ➤ Cooking Time: 10 minutes
> ➤ Servings: 4
> ➤ Level of difficulty: Easy

Ingredients:

- 11 oz sardines, canned, drained
- 1/3 cup shallot, chopped
- 1 teaspoon chili flakes
- ½ teaspoon salt
- 2 tablespoon corn flour
- 1 egg, beaten
- 1 tablespoon chives, chopped
- 1 teaspoon olive oil
- 1 teaspoon grass-fed butter

Directions:

1. Put the butter in the skillet and dissolve it. Add shallot and cook it until translucent. After this, transfer the shallot to the mixing bowl.

2. Add sardines, chili flakes, salt, flour, egg, chives, and mix up until smooth with the fork's help. Make the medium size cakes and place them in the skillet. Add olive oil.

3. Roast the fish cakes for 3 minutes from each side over medium heat. Dry the cooked fish cakes with a paper towel if needed and transfer them to the serving plates.

Nutrition:

Calories 221

Fat 12.2

Carbs 5.4

Protein 21.3

Grilled Catfish Fillets

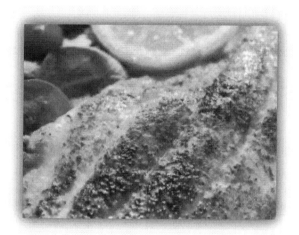

➤ Preparation Time: 10 minutes
➤ Cooking Time: 10 minutes
➤ Servings: 4
➤ Level of difficulty: Normal

Ingredients:

- 16 oz catfish steaks (4 oz each fish steak)
- 4 tbsp olive oil
- 1 squeezed lemon
- Salt and pepper as necessary

- 2 bay leaves
- ½ cup of breadcrumbs

Directions:

1. 1 Place the fish (without head and cut up to the tail) in marinade of oil, lemon, salt and pepper and two bay leaves, about 2 hours.
2. 2 Remove from marinade, pass in breadcrumbs, place on grill, sprinkle only initially, the fish with its marinade and let cook until golden brown.

Nutrition:

Calories 280

Fat 12

Carbs 6

Protein 21

4-Ingredients Salmon Fillet

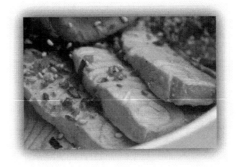

- ➢ Preparation Time: 5 minutes
- ➢ Cooking Time: 25 minutes
- ➢ Servings:1
- ➢ Level of difficulty: Normal

Ingredients:

- 8 oz salmon fillet
- ½ teaspoon salt
- 1 teaspoon sesame oil
- 1 teaspoon sesame seeds
- ½ teaspoon sage

Directions:

1. Rub the fillet with salt and sage. Put the fish in the tray, then sprinkle it with sesame oil. Cook the fish for 25 minutes at 365F. Flip the fish carefully onto another side after 12 minutes of cooking. Serve.

Nutrition:

Calories 161

Fat 11.6

Carbs 0.2

Protein 22

Cod Shakshuka Style

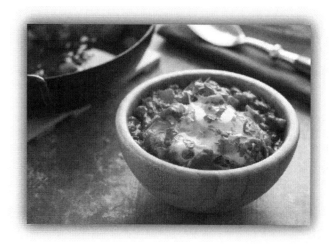

➢ Preparation Time: 5 minutes

➢ Cooking Time: 15 minutes

➢ Servings: 5

➢ Level of difficulty: Normal

Ingredients:

- 250 gr of cod fillet
- 5 eggs
- 1 cup tomatoes, chopped
- peppers, chopped
- 1 tablespoon ghee
- 1 teaspoon of tomato paste
- 1 teaspoon chili peppers
- 1 teaspoon whole sea salt
- 1 tablespoon fresh dill
- 1 tablespoon shallot, chopped

Directions:

1. Melt ghee in a saucepan and add chili, bell peppers and tomatoes. Sprinkle vegetables with shallots, dill, salt and chili. Simmer on low heat for 5 minutes.

2. Then add the chopped cod fillet and mix well. Close the lid and cook for 5 minutes over medium heat.

3. Finally crack the eggs over the fish and close the lid. Cook the Shakshuka with the pan covered for 5 minutes. Serve gently in deep bowls and enjoy hot.

Nutrition:

Calories 143

Fat 7.3

Carb. 7.9

Protein 12.8

Crazy Lamb Salad

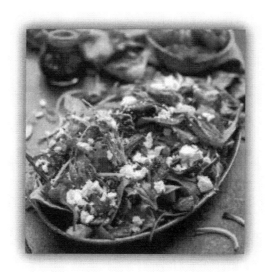

➤ Preparation time: 10 minutes
➤ Cooking Time: 35 minutes
➤ Servings: 4
➤ Level of difficulty: Normal

Ingredients:

- 1 tablespoon olive oil
- 1,5 -pound leg of lamb, bone removed, leg butterflied

- Salt and pepper to taste
- 1 teaspoon cumin
- Pinch of dried thyme
- 2 garlic cloves, peeled and minced

For Salad:

- 4 ounces feta cheese, crumbled
- ½ cup pecans
- 2 cups spinach
- 1 ½ tablespoon lemon juice
- ¼ cup olive oil
- 1 cup fresh mint, chopped

Directions:

1. Rub lamb with salt and pepper, 1 tablespoon oil, thyme, cumin, minced garlic. Preheat your grill to medium-high and transfer lamb.

2. Cook for 40 minutes, making sure to flip it once. Take a lined baking sheet and spread the pecans. Toast in oven for 10 minutes at 350-degree F.

3. Transfer grilled lamb to cutting board and let it cool, then slice after.

4. Take a salad bowl and add spinach, 1 cup mint, feta cheese, ¼ cup olive oil, lemon juice, toasted pecans, salt, pepper, and toss well. Add lamb slices on top. Serve.

Nutrition:

Calories: 334

Fat: 33g

Carbohydrates: 5g

Protein: 7g

Hearty Roasted Cauliflower

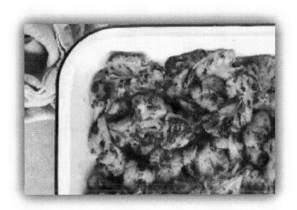

- ➢ Preparation time: 5 minutes
- ➢ Cooking Time: 30 minutes
- ➢ Servings: 8
- ➢ Level of difficulty: Normal

Ingredients:

- 1 large cauliflower head
- 2 tablespoons melted coconut oil
- 2 tablespoons fresh thyme
- 1 teaspoon Celtic sea sunflower seeds
- 1 teaspoon fresh ground pepper
- 1 head roasted garlic
- 2 tablespoons fresh thyme for garnish

Directions:

1. Warm your oven to 425 degrees F. Rinse cauliflower and trim, core, and slice. Lay cauliflower evenly on a rimmed baking tray.

2. Drizzle coconut oil evenly over cauliflower, sprinkle thyme leaves—season with a pinch of sunflower seeds and pepper. Squeeze roasted garlic.

3. Roast cauliflower until slightly caramelized for about 30 minutes, making sure to turn once. Garnish with fresh thyme leaves. Enjoy!

Nutrition:

Calories: 129

Fat: 11g

Carbohydrates: 6g

Protein: 7g

Cool Cabbage Fried Beef

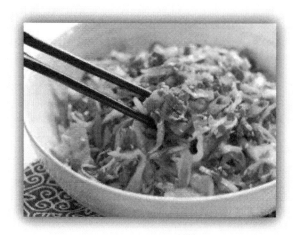

➤ Preparation time: 5 minutes
➤ Cooking Time: 15 minutes
➤ Servings: 4
➤ Level of difficulty: Normal

Ingredients:

- 1-pound beef, ground and lean
- ½ pound bacon
- 1 onion
- 1 garlic clove, minced
- ½ head cabbage
- Pepper to taste

Directions:

1. Take a skillet, then put it over medium heat. Add chopped bacon, beef, and onion until slightly browned. Move it to a bowl and keep it covered.

2. Add minced garlic and cabbage to the skillet and cook until slightly browned. Return the ground beef mixture to the skillet and simmer for 3-5 minutes over low heat. Serve and enjoy!

Nutrition:

Calories: 260

Fat: 12g

Carbohydrates: 5g

Protein: 24g

Fennel and Figs Lamb

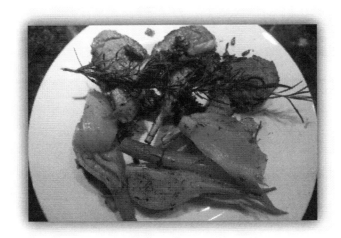

➢ Preparation time: 10 minutes
➢ Cooking Time: 40 minutes
➢ Servings: 2

> ➤ Level of difficulty: Normal

Ingredients:

- 7 ounces lamb racks
- 1 fennel bulbs, sliced
- 1 rosemary sprig
- pepper to taste
- 1 tablespoon olive oil
- 2 figs, cut in half
- 1/8 cup apple cider vinegar
- 1/2 tablespoon Erythritol

Directions:

1. Take a bowl and add fennel, figs, vinegar, Erythritol, oil, and toss. Transfer to baking dish. Season with sunflower seeds and pepper.

2. Bake within 15 minutes at 400 degrees F. Season lamb with sunflower seeds and pepper and transfer to a heated pan over medium-high heat. Cook for a few minutes.

3. Add lamb to the baking dish with fennel and bake for 20 minutes. Divide between plates and serve.

Nutrition:

Calories: 230

Fat: 3g

Carbohydrates: 5g

Protein: 10g

Mushroom and Olive "Mediterranean" Steak

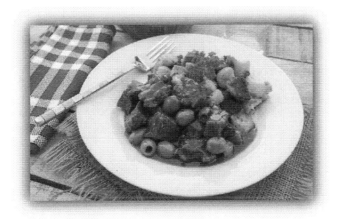

- ➢ Preparation time: 10 minutes
- ➢ Cooking Time: 14 minutes
- ➢ Servings: 2
- ➢ Level of difficulty: Normal

Ingredients:

- 1/2-pound boneless beef sirloin steak, ¾ inch thick, cut into 4 pieces
- 1/2 large red onion, chopped
- 1/2 cup mushrooms
- 2 garlic cloves, thinly sliced
- 2 tablespoons olive oil
- 1/4 cup green olives, coarsely chopped
- 1/2 cup parsley leaves, finely cut

Directions:

1. Take a large-sized skillet and place it over medium-high heat. Add oil and let it heat up. Add beef and cook until both sides are browned, remove beef and drain fat.

2. Add the rest of the oil to the skillet and heat. Add onions, garlic and cook for 2-3 minutes. Stir well. Add mushrooms, olives and cook until the mushrooms are thoroughly done.

3. Return the beef to the skillet, then adjust heat to medium. Cook for 3-4 minutes (covered). Stir in parsley. Serve and enjoy!

Nutrition:

Calories: 386

Fat: 30g

Carbohydrates: 11g

Protein: 21g

Chinese Style Spicy Chicken & Rice

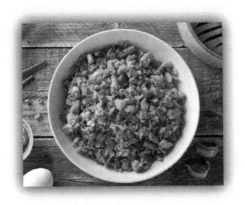

- ➢ Preparation time: 10 minutes
- ➢ Cooking Time: 12 minutes
- ➢ Servings: 4
- ➢ Level of difficulty: Easy

Ingredients:

- 1 teaspoon olive oil
- 4 large egg whites
- 1 onion, chopped
- 2 garlic cloves, minced
- 12 ounces skinless chicken breasts, boneless, cut into ½ inch cubes
- ½ cup carrots, chopped
- ½ cup of frozen green peas
- 2 cups long-grain brown rice, cooked

- 3 tablespoons soy sauce, low sodium

Directions:

1. Coat skillet with oil, place it over medium-high heat. Add egg whites and cook until scrambled. Sauté onion, garlic, and chicken breasts for 6 minutes.

2. Add carrots, peas and keep cooking for 3 minutes. Stir in rice, season with soy sauce. Add cooked egg whites, stir for 3 minutes. Enjoy!

Nutrition:

Calories: 323

Fat: 11g

Carbohydrates: 30g

Protein: 23g

Snack and Sides Recipes

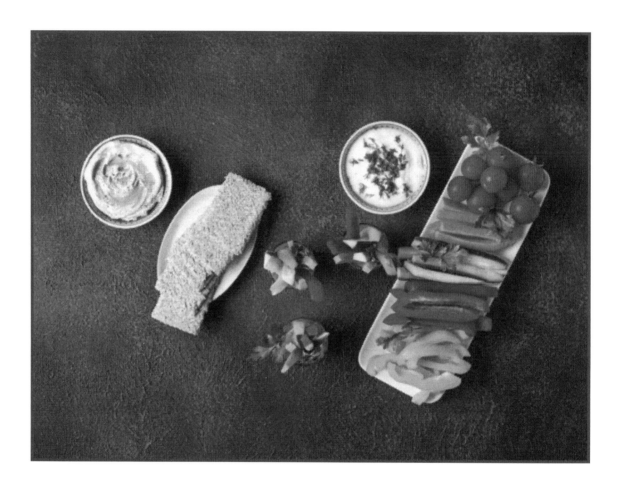

Cabbage Apple Stir-Fry

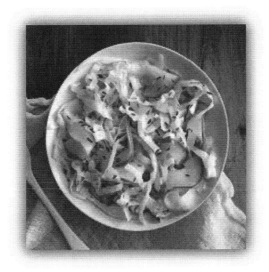

- ➢ Preparation Time: 15 Minutes
- ➢ Cooking Time: 10 Minutes
- ➢ Servings: 4
- ➢ Level of difficulty: Easy

Ingredients:

- 2 tablespoons extra-virgin olive oil
- 3 cups chopped cabbage
- 2 tablespoons water
- 1 Granny Smith apple, chopped
- 3 scallions, both white & green parts, chopped
- 3 tbsp olive oil
- 1 tbsp freshly squeezed lemon juice
- 1 teaspoon caraway seeds
- Pinch of salt

Directions:

1. In a big skillet or frying pan, heat the olive oil over medium-high temperature. Add the cabbage and stir-fry for 2 minutes. Add the water, cover, and cook for 2 minutes.

2. Uncover and stir in the apple and scallions and sprinkle with the lemon juice, caraway seeds, and salt—Stir-fry for 4 to 6 minutes longer, or until the cabbage is crisp-tender. Serve.

Nutrition:

Calories 106

Fat 7g

Carbohydrates 11g

Protein 1g

Parmesan Roasted Cauliflower

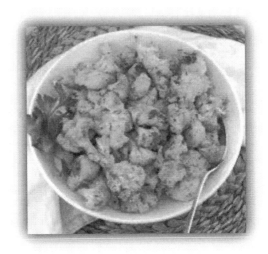

➢ Preparation Time: 15 Minutes
➢ Cooking Time: 25 Minutes
➢ Servings: 4
➢ Level of difficulty: Easy

Ingredients:

- 4 cups cauliflower florets
- ½ cup grated Parmesan cheese

- 2 tablespoons extra-virgin olive oil
- 4 garlic cloves, minced
- ½ teaspoon dried thyme leaves
- ¼ teaspoon freshly ground black pepper
- 1/8 teaspoon salt

Directions:

1. Preheat the oven to 400°F. On a baking sheet, combine the cauliflower, Parmesan cheese, olive oil, garlic, thyme, pepper, salt, and toss to coat.
2. Roast within 25 to 30 minutes, stirring once during cooking time, until the cauliflower has light golden-brown edges and is tender. Serve.

Nutrition:

Calories 144

Fat 11g

Carbohydrates 4g

Protein 6g

Celery and Fennel Salad with Cranberries

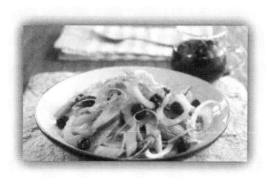

- ➤ Preparation Time: 15 Minutes
- ➤ Servings: 6
- ➤ Level of difficulty: Easy

Ingredients:

- ¼ cup extra-virgin olive oil
- 2 tablespoons freshly squeezed lemon juice
- 1 tablespoon Dijon mustard
- 2 cups sliced celery
- ½ cup chopped fennel
- ½ cup dried cranberries
- 2 tablespoons minced celery leaves
- lemon peels cut into strands

Directions:

1. In a serving bowl, whisk the olive oil, lemon juice, and mustard. Add the celery, fennel, and cranberries to the dressing and toss to coat.
2. Sprinkle with the lemon peels and serve.

Nutrition:

Calories 130

Fat 9g

Carbohydrates 13g

Protein <1g

Kale with Caramelized Onions

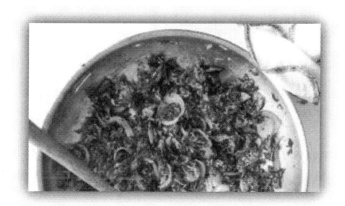

- ➢ Preparation Time: 15 Minutes
- ➢ Cooking Time: 20 Minutes
- ➢ Servings: 4
- ➢ Level of difficulty: Normal

Ingredients:

- • 1 bunch green kale, rinsed and torn into pieces
- • 1 yellow onion, chopped
- • 2 tablespoons grass-fed butter
- • 1 tablespoon extra-virgin olive oil
- • 2 tablespoons water
- • 1 tablespoon freshly squeezed lemon juice
- • 1 teaspoon maple syrup
- • Whole sea salt
- • Freshly ground black pepper

Directions:

1. In a heavy saucepan, combine the onion, butter, and olive oil over medium heat. Cook for about 3 minutes, until the onion starts to become translucent, stirring frequently.

2. Adjust the heat to low, then cook for 10 to 15 minutes longer, frequently stirring, until the onion starts to brown.

3. Adjust the heat again to medium and add the kale and water. Cover the pan and cook for about 2 minutes, shaking the pan occasionally, until the kale starts to soften.

4. Put the lemon juice plus maple syrup, and season with salt plus pepper. Cook within 3 to 4 minutes longer, frequently stirring until the kale is tender. Serve.

Nutrition:

Calories 115

Fat 10g

Carbohydrates 6g

Protein 2g

Italian Peas and Mint Risotto

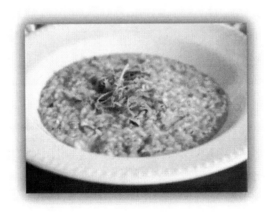

➢ Preparation Time: 10 Minutes
➢ Cooking Time: 35 Minutes
➢ Servings: 4
➢ Level of difficulty: Normal

Ingredients:

- 2 tablespoons extra-virgin olive oil

- 1 onion, chopped

- 12 oz of brown rice

- 1/8 teaspoon salt

- 2½ cups water, divided

- 2 cups frozen baby peas

- ¼ teaspoon dried mint leaves

- 2 tablespoons grated Parmesan cheese

Directions:

1. Heat-up olive oil over medium heat in a large saucepan. Put the onion and cook within 2 to 3 minutes, stirring, until tender.
2. Put the rice, then stir and sprinkle with the salt.
3. Add 1 cup of water; cook for 5 to 10 minutes, stirring, until the water is absorbed.
4. Add another ½ cup of water; cook and stir until it's absorbed, approximately for another 5 minutes. Then add the remaining 1 cup of water, cover the pan
5. Simmer for about 20 minutes, occasionally stirring, until the rice is tender. Using this method will force the rice to omit some starch as it cooks, making the dish creamier.
6. Put the peas plus mint in the pan. Cook within 3 to 5 minutes, frequently stirring until the peas are hot and tender. Sprinkle with the cheese and serve.

Nutrition:

Calories 317

Fat 10g

Carbohydrates 50g

Protein 9g

Spicy Baked Sweet Potato Wedges

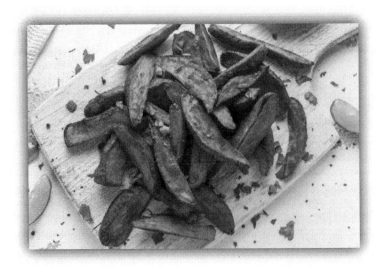

- ➢ Preparation time: 20 minutes
- ➢ Cooking time: 45 minutes
- ➢ Servings: 4
- ➢ Level of difficulty: Normal

Ingredients:

- 450 g sweet potatoes
- 1 tablespoon of ghee
- 1 tablespoon extra virgin olive oil
- 1 teaspoon of chili powder
- 1 teaspoon of paprika
- ¼ teaspoon salt
- 1/8 teaspoon freshly ground black pepper
- 1 tablespoon chopped parsley
- lime wedges

Directions:

1. Peel the potatoes and cut into slices.
2. Preheat oven to 375F.

3.   Melt the ghee with the olive oil in a small saucepan. Drizzle the potatoes with this dressing on a baking sheet lined with baking paper. Sprinkle with the chili powder, paprika, salt and pepper and toss to coat. Spread the strips in a single layer.

4.   Bake the potatoes for 40-45 minutes or until golden brown and crisp, turning once with a spatula halfway through the cooking time. Sprinkle with parsley and serve with lime wedges.

Nutrition:

Calories 180

Fat 10g

Carb. 11g

Protein 2g

Delicious Veggies in Apple Cider Vinegar

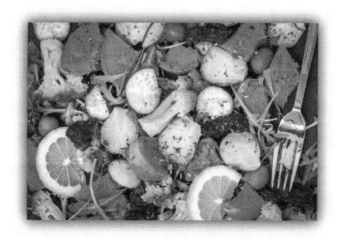

➢ Preparation time: 20 minutes
➢ Cooking time: 25 minutes
➢ Servings: 4
➢ Level of difficulty: Normal

Ingredients:

- 1 sweet potato peeled and cut into chunks
- 150 gr of broccoli

- 1 cup radishes
- 1 cup Brussels sprouts
- ½ cup sun-dried tomatoes
- ½ cup green olives
- 250 g arugula
- ½ lemon in thin slices
- tablespoons of extra virgin olive oil
- 1 tablespoon apple cider vinegar
- 1 pinch of salt
- 1 pinch of freshly ground black pepper

Directions:

1. Fill a large casserole dish halfway, and place a multi-level steamer basket on top, where you will cook the broccoli, Brussels sprouts and sweet potato.
2. Cook for 20 minutes. Remove from heat and allow to cool.
3. Meanwhile, soak the sun-dried tomatoes, cut the radishes into thin slices, and wash the arugula.
4. Make a vinaigrette with the oil, apple cider vinegar, salt and pepper and mix quickly with a fork.
5. Prepare a salad bowl, and pour in all the steamed vegetables, cut radishes, drained and chopped sun-dried tomatoes, olives, and arugula.
6. Dress with the vinaigrette and serve.

Nutrition:

Calories 86

Fats 10 g

Carbs 29 g

Protein 1 g

Roasted Onion Dip

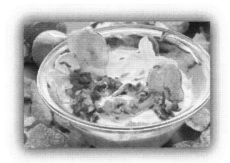

➢ Preparation time: 15 minutes

➢ Cooking time: 35 minutes

➢ Servings: 1 cup

➢ Level of difficulty: Easy

Ingredients:

- 1 red onion, chopped

- 2 tablespoons extra-virgin olive oil

- 1 package cream cheese, at room temperature

- 2 tablespoons mayonnaise (homemade with olive oil)

- 1 tablespoon freshly squeezed lemon juice

- ½ teaspoon dried thyme leaves

Directions:

1. Preheat the oven to 400°F. Mix the onion and olive oil and toss to coat on a rimmed baking sheet.

2. Roast for 30 to 35 minutes, occasionally stirring until the onions are soft and golden brown. Don't let them burn. Transfer to a plate and set aside.

3. Beat the cream cheese, mayonnaise, lemon juice, and thyme leaves on a rimmed baking sheet. Stir in the onions. Serve the dip at this point or cover and refrigerate it up to 8 hours before serving.

Nutrition:

Calories 212

Fat 21g

Carbohydrates 4g

Protein 3g

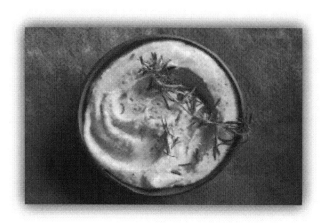

Roasted Garlic White Bean Dip

- ➢ Preparation time: 20 minutes
- ➢ Cooking time: 60 minutes
- ➢ Servings: 2
- ➢ Level of difficulty: Normal

Ingredients:

- 2 onions, cut into 8 wedges each
- 2 garlic heads, whole
- ¼ cup extra-virgin olive oil, divided
- 1 (15-ounce) can no-salt-added cannellini beans, drained and rinsed
- 2 tablespoons freshly squeezed lemon juice
- 1 teaspoon dried marjoram leaves
- 1/8 teaspoon salt

- 1/8 teaspoon freshly ground black pepper

Directions:

1. Preheat the oven to 375°F. On a rimmed baking sheet, place the onions. Cut the top inch off each garlic head, just enough to expose the cloves, and discard the top.

2. Place the garlic, with the exposed cloves facing up, on the baking sheet. Drizzle 1 tablespoon of olive oil directly into the garlic heads.

3. Wrap each head in aluminum foil and place back on the baking sheet. Drizzle the onions with another 1 tablespoon of olive oil.

4. Roast the vegetables for 45 to 55 minutes, stirring the onions once during cooking.

5. Remove the foil from the garlic and let the garlic and onions cool for 30 minutes. Blend the cannellini beans, lemon juice, marjoram, salt, and pepper in a blender or food processor.

6. Add the onions. Squeeze the garlic head, so the cloves pop out, and add to the blender.

7. Blend or process the mixture, drizzling in the remaining 2 tablespoons of olive oil, until it is mostly smooth, with some texture. Serve.

Nutrition:

Calories 166

Fat 10g

Carbohydrates 17g

Protein 4g

Green Goddess Dip

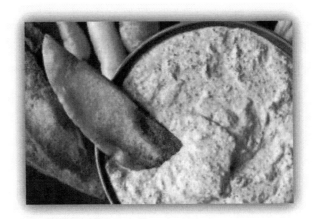

- ➢ Preparation time: 15 minutes
- ➢ Servings: 1 bowl
- ➢ Level of difficulty: Easy

Ingredients:

- 1 package cream cheese, at room temperature
- 3 tablespoons freshly squeezed lemon juice
- 2 teaspoons Worcestershire sauce
- ½ cup chopped flat-leaf parsley
- ¼ cup minced fresh chives

Directions:

1. Mix the cream cheese, lemon juice, and Worcestershire sauce in a medium bowl, and beat until smooth.

2. Stir in the parsley and chives. You can serve the dip immediately or cover and chill for 4 to 6 hours before serving.

Nutrition:

Calories 139

Fat 13g

Carbohydrates 4g

Protein 3g

Crab and Carrot Dip

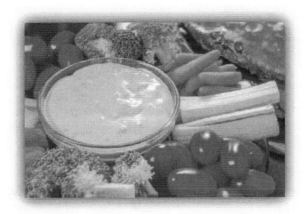

- ➢ Preparation time: 20 minutes
- ➢ Servings: 1 ½ cups
- ➢ Level of difficulty: Easy

Ingredients:

- 1 cup mascarpone cheese
- 2 tablespoons freshly squeezed lemon juice
- ½ cup lump crab meat, drained
- 1 cup grated carrots
- 4 scallions, both green & white parts, chopped

Directions:

1. Beat the mascarpone and lemon juice until smooth in a medium bowl. Look over the crab, removing any bits of cartilage and discarding.

2. Stir the crab, carrots, and scallions into the mascarpone mixture. Serve.

Nutrition:

Calories 194

Fat 18g

Carbohydrates 4g

Protein 5g

Baba Ghanoush

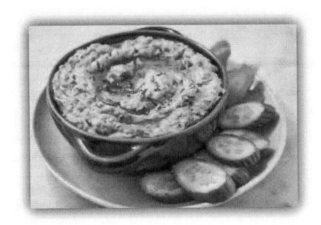

- ➤ Preparation Time: 20 minutes
- ➤ Cooking Time: 30 minutes
- ➤ Servings: 6
- ➤ Level of difficulty: Normal

Ingredients:

- 1 eggplant, halved and scored with a crosshatch pattern on the cut sides
- 1 tbsp olive oil, + extra for brushing
- 1 sweet onion, peeled and diced
- 2 cloves garlic, halved
- 2 tsp ground cumin
- 1 tsp ground coriander
- 1 tbsp lemon juice
- freshly ground black pepper

Directions:

1. Preheat the oven to 400F. Line 2 baking sheets with parchment paper. Brush the eggplant halves using the olive oil and place them, cut side down, on 1 baking sheet.

2. Mix the onion, garlic, 1 tbsp olive oil, cumin, plus coriander in a small bowl. Spread the seasoned onions on the other baking sheet.

3. Put both baking sheets in your oven. Roast the onions for about 20 minutes and the eggplant for 30 minutes, or until softened and browned.

4. Remove the vegetables, then scrape the eggplant flesh into a bowl. Move the onions plus garlic to a cutting board and chop coarsely; add to the eggplant.

5. Stir in the lemon juice and pepper. Serve warm or chilled.

Nutrition:

Calories: 45

Fat: 2g

Carb: 6g

Protein: 1g

Spicy Kale Chips

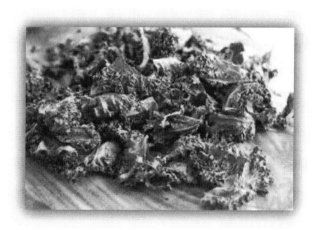

➢ Preparation Time: 20 minutes
➢ Cooking Time: 25 minutes
➢ Servings: 6
➢ Level of difficulty: Normal

Ingredients:

- 2 cups kale
- 2 tsp olive oil
- ¼ tsp chili powder
- pinch cayenne pepper

Directions:

1. Preheat the oven to 300F. Discard the stems from your kale and tear the leaves into 2-inch pieces.
2. Wash the kale and dry it thoroughly. Move the kale to a large bowl and drizzle with olive oil. Use your hands to toss the kale with oil, taking care to coat each leaf evenly.
3. Season the kale with chili powder and cayenne pepper and toss to combine thoroughly. Spread the seasoned kale in a single layer on each baking sheet. Do not overlap the leaves.
4. Brown, preferably in a ventilated oven, rotating the pans once, for 20-25 minutes until it is crisp and dry. Remove the trays, then allow the chips cool on the pans for 5 minutes. Serve.

Nutrition:

Calories: 24   Fat: 2g

Carb: 2g   Protein: 1g

Cinnamon Tortilla Chips

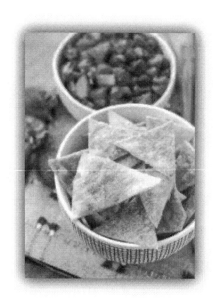

- ➤ Preparation Time: 15 minutes
- ➤ Cooking Time: 10 minutes
- ➤ Servings: 6

> Level of difficulty: Easy

Ingredients:

- 2 tsp brown sugar
- ½ tsp ground cinnamon
- pinch ground nutmeg
- 3 kamut tortillas
- Ghee for oiling

Directions:

1. Preheat the oven to 350F. Line a baking sheet with parchment paper. Mix the sugar, cinnamon, plus nutmeg in a small bowl.
2. Lay the tortillas on your clean work surface and spray both sides of each lightly with ghee. Sprinkle the cinnamon sugar evenly over both sides of each tortilla.
3. Cut the tortillas into 16 wedges each and place them on the baking sheet. Bake the tortilla wedges, turning once, for about 10 minutes or until crisp. Cool the chips. Serve.

Nutrition:

Calories: 51

Fat: 1g

Carb: 9g

Protein: 1g

Sweet and Spicy Kettle Corn

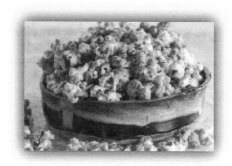

> ➢ Preparation Time: 1 minute
> ➢ Cooking Time: 5 minutes
> ➢ Servings: 8
> ➢ Level of difficulty: Easy

Ingredients:

- 3 tbsp olive oil
- 1 cup popcorn kernels
- ½ cup brown sugar
- pinch cayenne pepper

Directions:

1. Put a large pot with a lid on medium heat and add the olive oil with a few popcorn kernels. Shake the pot lightly until the popcorn kernels pop. Put the rest of the kernels and sugar in the pot.

2. Pop the kernels with the lid on the pot, continually shaking, until they are popped. Remove the pot, then put the popcorn in a large bowl. Toss the popcorn with the cayenne pepper and serve.

Nutrition:

Calories: 186

Fat: 6g

Carb: 30g

Protein: 3g

Meringue Cookies

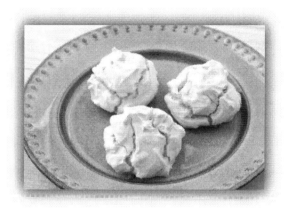

- ➤ Preparation Time: 30 minutes
- ➤ Cooking Time: 30 minutes
- ➤ Servings: 24
- ➤ Level of difficulty: Normal

Ingredients:

- 4 egg whites
- 1 cup Erythritol
- 1 tsp pure vanilla extract
- 1 tsp almond extract

Directions:

1. Preheat the oven to 300F. Line 2 baking sheets with parchment paper. Set aside. Beat your egg whites until soft peaks.
2. Blend the erythritol in a grinder a little at a time and reduce to a powder.

3. Put the Erythritol 1 tbsp at a time. Beat well to mix after each addition. The meringue should be thick and glossy.
4. Beat in the vanilla extract plus almond extract. Using a tbsp, drop the meringue batter onto the baking sheets, spacing the cookies evenly.
5. Bake the cookies within 30 minutes, or until they are crisp. Remove the cookies, then let it cool on wire racks. Serve.

Nutrition:

Calories: 36

Fat: 0g

Carb: 8g

Protein: 1g

Corn Bread

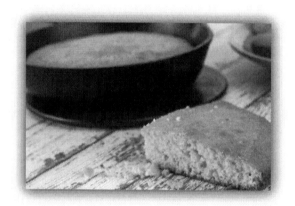

- ➢ Preparation Time: 10 minutes
- ➢ Cooking Time: 20 minutes
- ➢ Servings: 10
- ➢ Level of difficulty: Normal

Ingredients:

- Olive oil for greasing the baking dish
- 1 ¼ cups of organic no GMO cornmeal
- ¾ cup rice flour
- 1 tbsp cream of tartar yeast
- ½ cup Erythritol
- 2 eggs
- 1 cup unsweetened, unfortified rice milk
- 2 tbsp olive oil

Directions:

1. Preheat the oven to 425F. Oiled 8-by-8-inch baking dish with olive oil. Set aside. Mix the cornmeal, rice flour, cream of tartar yeast, and Erythritol in a medium bowl.
2. Mix the eggs, rice milk, and olive oil until blended in a small bowl. Put the wet fixings to the dry ingredients and stir until well combined.
3. Put the batter into your baking dish and bake within 20 minutes or until golden and cooked through. Serve warm.

Nutrition:

Calories: 198

Fat: 5g

Carb: 34g

Protein: 4g

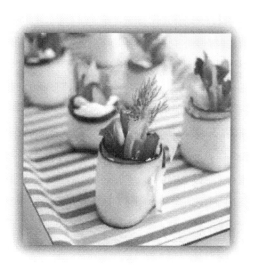

Cucumber-Wrapped Vegetable Rolls

- ➢ Preparation Time: 30 minutes
- ➢ Servings: 8
- ➢ Level of difficulty: Easy

Ingredients:

- ½ cup finely shredded red cabbage
- ½ cup grated carrot
- ¼ cup julienne red bell pepper
- ¼ cup julienned scallion, both green and white parts
- ¼ cup chopped cilantro
- 1 tbsp olive oil
- ¼ tsp ground cumin
- ¼ tsp freshly ground black pepper
- 1 English cucumber, sliced into skinny strips

Directions:

1. In a bowl, toss together the black pepper, cumin, olive oil, cilantro, scallion, red pepper, carrot, and cabbage. Mix well.
2. Evenly divide the vegetable filling among the cucumber strips, placing the filling close to one end of the strip.
3. Roll up the cucumber strips around the filling and secure with a wooden pick. Repeat with each cucumber strip. Serve.

Nutrition:

Calories: 26

Fat: 2g

Carb: 3g

Protein: 0g

Chicken, Pumpkin and Onion Skewers

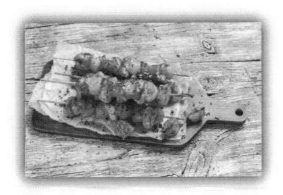

- ➢ Preparation Time: 15 minutes
- ➢ Cooking Time: 12 minutes
- ➢ Servings: 4
- ➢ Level of difficulty: Easy

Ingredients:

- 2 tbsp olive oil
- 2 tbsp freshly squeezed lemon juice
- ½ tsp minced garlic
- ½ tsp chopped fresh thyme
- 6 oz chicken breast, boneless & skinless cut into 8 pieces
- 1 small summer squash, cut into 8 pieces
- ½ medium onion, cut into 8 pieces

Directions:

1. Mix the olive oil, lemon juice, garlic, and thyme in a bowl. Put the chicken in the bowl, then mix to coat.
2. Wrap the bowl with plastic wrap and place the chicken in the refrigerator to marinate for 1 hour.
3. Thread the squash, onion, and chicken pieces onto 4 large skewers, evenly dividing the vegetable and meat among the skewers.
4. Heat-up barbecue to medium and grill the skewers, turning at least 2 times, for 10 to 12 minutes.

Nutrition:

Calories: 106

Fat: 8g

Carb: 3g

Protein: 7g

Chicken Lettuce Wraps

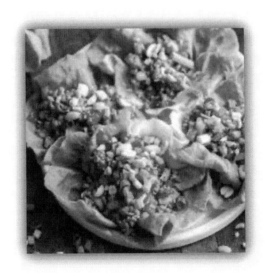

- ➢ Preparation Time: 30 minutes
- ➢ Servings: 8
- ➢ Level of difficulty: Easy

Ingredients:

- 6 oz Cooked chicken breast, minced
- 1 Scallion, both green and white parts, chopped
- ½ Red apple, cored and chopped
- ½ cup Bean sprouts
- ¼ English cucumber, chopped

- Juice of 1 lime

- Zest of 1 lime

- 2 tbsp Chopped fresh cilantro

- ½ tsp Chinese five-spice powder

- 8 Boston lettuce leaves

Directions:

1. In a bowl, mix the scallions, chicken, apple, cucumber, bean sprouts, lime juice, lime zest, cilantro, plus five-spice powder.

2. Mix together the chopped chicken, and place evenly on the 8 lettuce leaves, in serving dishes. Serve immediately.

Nutrition:

Calories: 51

Fat: 2g

Carb: 2g

Protein: 7g

Antojitos

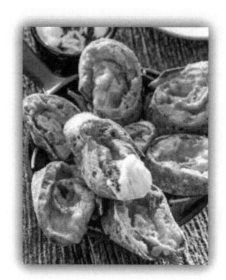

- ➢ Preparation Time: 20 minutes
- ➢ Servings: 8
- ➢ Level of difficulty: Easy

Ingredients:

- 6 oz plain cream cheese
- ½ jalapeno pepper, finely chopped
- ½ scallion, green part only, chopped
- ¼ cup finely chopped red bell pepper
- ½ tsp ground cumin
- ½ tsp ground coriander
- ½ tsp chili powder
- 3 kamut or buckwheat tortillas, (8-inch)

Directions:

1. In a bowl, mix the jalapeno pepper, cream cheese, scallion, red bell pepper, cumin, coriander, and chili powder until well blended.

2. Split the cream cheese mixture evenly on the 3 tortillas, spreading the cheese in a thin layer and leaving a ¼ inch edge all the way around.

3. Roll the tortillas like a jelly roll and wrap each tightly in plastic wrap. Refrigerate the rolls for about 1 hour or until they are set. Cut the rolls and serve.

Nutrition:

Calories: 110

Fat: 8g

Carb: 7g

Protein: 2g

Roasted Onion Garlic Dip

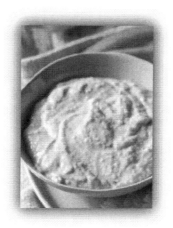

- ➢ Preparation Time: 15 minutes
- ➢ Cooking Time: 1 hour
- ➢ Servings: 6
- ➢ Level of difficulty: Normal

Ingredients:

- 1 sweet onion, peeled and cut into eights
- 8 cloves garlic
- 2 tsp olive oil
- ½ cup light sour cream
- 1 tbsp fresh lemon juice
- 1 tbsp chopped fresh parsley
- 1 tsp chopped fresh thyme
- ground black pepper

Directions:

1. Preheat the oven to 425F. Toss the onion and garlic in a bowl with olive oil. Transfer the onion and garlic to a piece of aluminum foil and wrap the vegetables loosely in a packet.

2. Put the foil packet on your small baking sheet and place the sheet in the oven. Roast the vegetables within 50 minutes to 1 hour, or until they are very fragrant and golden.

3. Remove the packet, then allow it to cool for 15 minutes. In a bowl, stir together the lemon juice, sour cream, parsley, thyme, and black pepper.

4. Open the foil packet carefully and transfer the vegetables to a cutting board. Chop the vegetables, then put it into the sour cream mixture. Stir to combine.

5. Cover the dip and chill in the refrigerator for 1 hour. Serve.

Nutrition:

Calories: 44

Fat: 3g

Carb: 5g

Protein: 1g

Cheese-Herb Dip

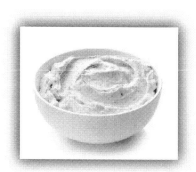

➤ Preparation Time: 20 minutes
➤ Servings: 8
➤ Level of difficulty: Easy

Ingredients:

- 1 cup cream cheese
- ½ cup unsweetened rice milk
- ½ scallion, green part only, chopped
- 1 tbsp chopped fresh parsley
- 1 tbsp chopped fresh basil
- 1 tbsp lemon juice
- 1 tsp minced garlic
- ½ tsp chopped fresh thyme
- ¼ tsp ground black pepper

Directions:

1. In a bowl, mix the milk, cream cheese, parsley, scallion, basil, lemon juice, garlic, thyme, and pepper until well combined. Store and use.

Nutrition:

Calories: 108

Fat: 10g

Carb: 3g

Protein: 2g

Zesty Chicken Wings

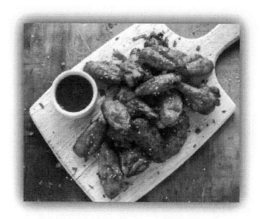

- ➤ Preparation time: 4-6 hours & 15 minutes
- ➤ Cooking time: 35 minutes
- ➤ Servings: 2
- ➤ Level of difficulty: Normal

Ingredients:

- 1 green onion, chopped
- ½ tablespoons reduced-sodium soy sauce
- ¼ tablespoon honey
- ¼ teaspoons allspice
- ¼ teaspoons dried thyme
- ½ teaspoon ginger
- ¼ teaspoon minced garlic
- 1/8 cup apple cider vinegar
- 1/8 cup lime juice
- 1/8 cup cranberry juice
- 1-pound chicken wings

Directions:

1. Mix all ingredients except the chicken wings. Set aside ¾ cup of marinade. Place duck wings into a container or large resealable plastic bag. Pour the extra marinade over wings.

2. Cover and marinate in the refrigerator within 4 to 6 hours—Preheat oven to 3500F. Place chicken wings on a baking sheet and bake for 20 minutes.

3. Meanwhile, in a small saucepan, bring reserved 3/4 cup marinade to a boil. Reduce by 1/3 until it thickens slightly to a glaze (approximately 10 minutes).

4. After 20 minutes, remove the chicken from the oven and brush the wings with the glaze. Raise oven temperature to 400F and cook chicken wings for about another 20 minutes, until done.

Nutrition:

Calories 78

Fat 2.6g

Carbohydrate 2.3g

Protein 10.4g

Yogurt Fruit Dip

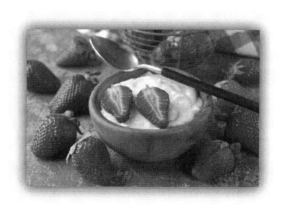

➢ Preparation time: 15 minutes
➢ Servings: 2
➢ Level of difficulty: Easy

Ingredients:

- 1-ounce light cream cheese
- 1-ounce low-fat Greek yogurt
- 1/4 cup strawberry

- 1 teaspoon cinnamon
- 1 tablespoon honey
- 2 drops of vanilla essence

Directions:

1. Mix ingredients with a hand mixer in a medium mixing bowl until smooth. Refrigerate until ready to serve.

Nutrition:

Calories 104

Fat 5.2g

Carbohydrate 14g

Protein 1.8g

Veggie Healthy Chips

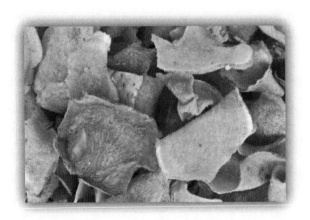

➢ Preparation time: 30 minutes
➢ Cooking time: 20 minutes
➢ Servings: 4/6
➢ Level of difficulty: Easy

Ingredients:

- 200 gr beet
- 150 gr sweet potatoes

- 150 gr carrots
- 2 zucchini
- q.b. salt
- q.b. pepper
- to taste spices
- to taste aromatic herbs

Directions:

1. Leave the skin on potatoes, zucchini, eggplant while other vegetables can have it removed. For potatoes, rinse them several times after cutting to remove the starch and then dry them with a clean cloth.
2. Cut the cleaned vegetables into thin strips or rounds, using a mandoline.
3. Arrange the vegetables in a single layer on the baking sheet, lined with baking paper or lightly greased. You can pass them in a mixture of extra virgin olive oil with a pinch of salt but it is not necessary. In any case, before baking them, sprinkle with some salt, herbs, spices according to what you like best.
4. To cook, bake the vegetables in the preheated ventilated oven at 160 degrees for about 20 minutes. Check, because depending on the type of vegetable, some cook earlier, others later. Serve in a bowl.

Nutrition:

Calories 282

Fat 13.5 g

Carb. 13.3 g

Protein 2.2 g

Roasted Grapes

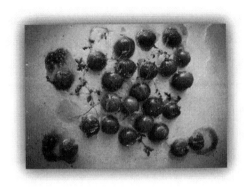

> ➢ Preparation time: 5 minutes
> ➢ Cooking time: 15 minutes
> ➢ Servings: 2
> ➢ Level of difficulty: Easy

Ingredients:

- 1-1/2 cups red or green grapes
- Olive oil
- ½ tablespoon chopped fresh thyme
- ½ tablespoon chopped fresh oregano
- Ground black pepper to taste
- ¼ teaspoon lemon juice

Directions:

1. Preheat oven to 375 degrees F. Mix grapes, olive oil, thyme, and oregano in a bowl and lightly toss to coat. Place grapes on a baking sheet.

2. Bake in the preheated oven until grapes begin to wrinkle and split, about 15 minutes. Drizzle with lemon juice and season with ground black pepper.

Nutrition:

Calories 56

Fat 4.9g

Carbohydrate 3.8g

Protein 0.5g

Spicy Strawberry Plums Peach Salsa

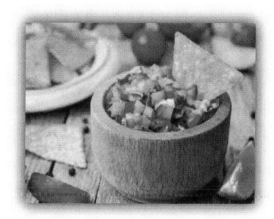

➢ Preparation time: 15 minutes

➢ Servings: 2

➢ Level of difficulty: Easy

Ingredients:

- 1 ripe peach - peeled, pitted, and diced
- 2 plums diced
- 2 fresh strawberries, diced
- ¼ jalapeno pepper, seeded and diced
- ½ tablespoon lime juice
- ¼ teaspoon honey
- ½ green onion, chopped
- 1 tablespoon chopped fresh cilantro

Directions:

1. Combine the peach, plums, strawberries, jalapeno pepper, lime juice, green onion, cilantro, and honey in a bowl; gently stir to combine. Serve.

Nutrition:

Calories 68

Fat 0.5g

Carbohydrate 17.2g

Protein 1.4g

Cucumber Pineapple Salsa

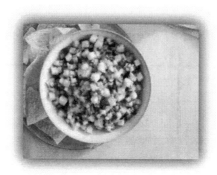

- ➢ Preparation time: 30 minutes
- ➢ Servings: 2
- ➢ Level of difficulty: Easy

Ingredients:

- ½ large cucumbers, finely diced
- 1/8 tablespoon extra-virgin olive oil
- ½ cup pineapple chucks
- 1/8 jalapeno pepper, seeded and minced
- ¼ lime, juiced and zest
- ¼ small red onion, chopped
- 1 bunch cilantro, coarsely chopped
- 1 pinch ground black pepper

Directions:

1. Mix the cucumbers, pineapple, olive oil, jalapeno pepper, lime juice, lime zest, red onion, cilantro, and pepper in a large serving bowl.
2. Wrap the bowl using a plastic wrap, and chill in the refrigerator for at least 2 hours to let the flavors blend. Serve.

Nutrition:

Calories 46

Fat 1.1g

Carbohydrate 10g

Protein 0.9g

Fruity Fun Skewers

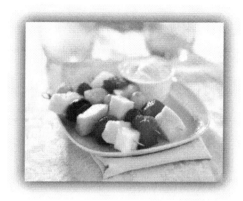

> ➢ Preparation time: 15 minutes
> ➢ Servings: 2
> ➢ Level of difficulty: Easy

Ingredients:

- 4 large strawberries, halved
- ¼ pineapple, peeled and cut into chunks
- 1 apple, cut into chunks
- 4 grapes
- 2 skewers

Directions:

1. Wash and dry the fruit.
2. Thread the strawberries, pineapple, grapes, plus apple pieces alternately onto skewers, placing at least 2 of the fruit on each skewer. Serve the fruit skewers decoratively on a serving platter.

Nutrition:

Calories 50

Fat 0.2g

Carbohydrate 13.3g

Protein 0.4g

Healthy, Delicious Dessert

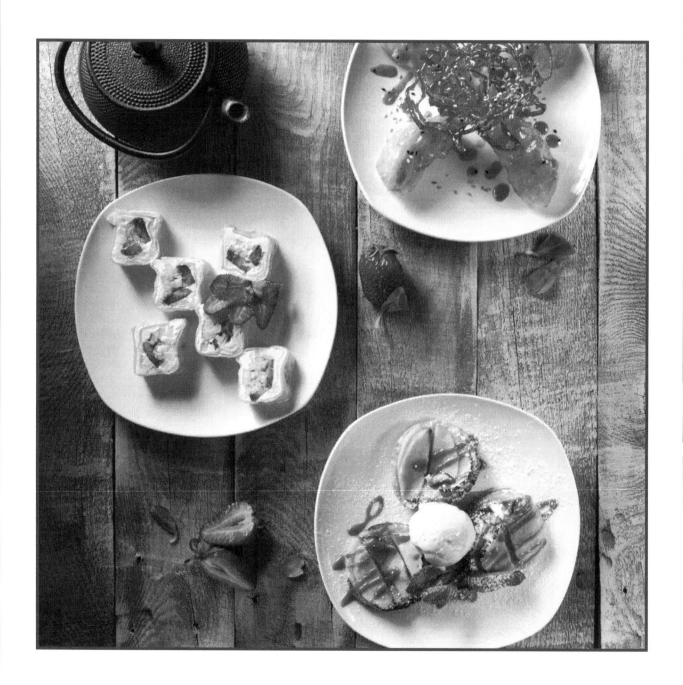

Grilled Peach Sundaes

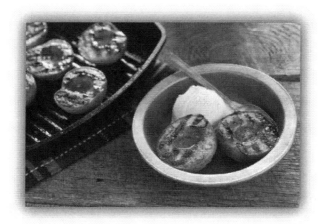

- ➢ Preparation time: 10 minutes
- ➢ Cooking time: 5 minutes
- ➢ Servings: 2
- ➢ Level of difficulty: Easy

Ingredients:

- 2 tbsp unsweetened coconut cream
- 1 teaspoon of ghee
- 4 peaches, cut in half and pitted
- 4 tbsp low-fat vanilla yogurt kept in the freezer

Directions:

1. Remove the yogurt from the freezer, and wait until it can be whipped up. Then combine it with the coconut.
2. Brush the peaches with the ghee and grill until tender. Place the peach halves in a bowl and add the yogurt whipped with the coconut.

Nutrition:

Calories: 61

Carbs: 2g

Protein: 2g

Fats: 6g

Blueberry Swirl Cake

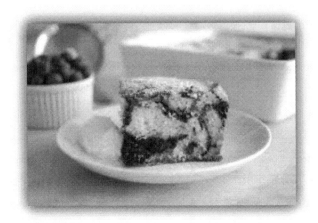

- ➤ Preparation time: 15 minutes
- ➤ Cooking time: 47 minutes
- ➤ Servings: 9
- ➤ Level of difficulty: Normal

Ingredients:

- ½ cup grass-fed unsalted butter
- 1 ¼ cups coconut milk
- 1 cup Erythritol
- 1 egg
- 1 egg white
- 1 tbsp lemon zest, grated
- 1 tsp cinnamon
- 1/3 cup light brown sugar
- 2 ½ cups fresh blueberries
- 2 ½ cups rice flour
- 1/2 bag of cream of tartar yeast

Directions:

1. Cream the butter and Erythritol using an electric mixer at high speed until fluffy. Add the egg and egg white and beat for another two minutes.
2. Add the lemon zest and reduce the speed to low. Add the rice flour with coconut milk alternately.

3. In a greased 13x19 pan, spread half of the batter and sprinkle with a half of blueberry. Add the remaining batter and blueberry on top. Bake in a 350-degree Fahrenheit preheated oven for 45 minutes. Serve.

Nutrition:

Calories: 284

Carbs: 43g

Protein: 7g

Fats: 13g

Peanut Butter Cookies

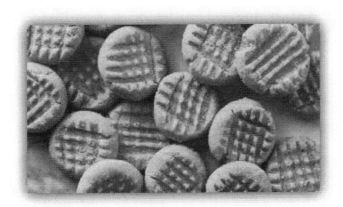

> ➤ Preparation time: 15 minutes
> ➤ Cooking time: 24 minutes
> ➤ Servings: 24
> ➤ Level of difficulty: Normal

Ingredients:

- ¼ cup Erythritol
- 1 cup unsalted peanut butter
- 1 tsp baking soda

- 2 cups almond flour
- 2 large eggs
- 2 tbsp grass-fed unsalted butter
- 2 tsp pure vanilla extract
- 4 ounces softened cream cheese

Directions:

1. Prepare a cookie sheet with a non-stick liner. Set aside. In a bowl, mix flour, Erythritol, and baking soda. Set aside. Mix the butter, cream cheese, and peanut butter in a mixing bowl.

2. Mix on high speed until it forms a smooth consistency. Put the eggs plus vanilla gradually while mixing until it forms a smooth texture.

3. Add the almond flour mixture slowly and mix until well combined.

4. Put the dough using a 1 tablespoon cookie scoop and drop each cookie on the prepared cookie sheet. Press the cookie with a fork and bake for 10 to 12 minutes at 350 F.

Nutrition:

Calories: 138

Carbs: 12g

Protein: 4g

Fats: 9g

Banana Foster

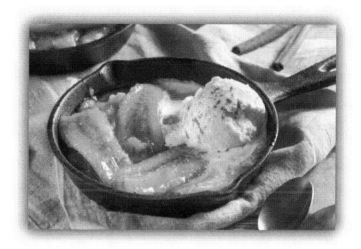

> ➤ Preparation time: 15 minutes
> ➤ Rest: 2 hours
> ➤ Cooking time: 5 minutes
> ➤ Servings: 8
> ➤ Level of difficulty: normal

Ingredients:

- ½ cup of Erythritol + 1 tbsp
- ½ cup melted coconut oil
- ½ teaspoon nutmeg
- ¾ cup cashew butter
- 1 tablespoon coconut oil
- 1/3 cup arrowroot starch
- 2 ¼ teaspoon dark rum
- 2 teaspoon cinnamons
- 2 teaspoon vanilla extract
- 3 cups coconut cream
- 4 ripe bananas, sliced

Directions:

1. In a bowl, whip the coconut cream until frothy. Add the arrowroot starch and whip for another minute. Very slowly add the cashew butter.

2. Stir in the erythritol, nutmeg and cinnamon and whip for another 2 minutes until the erythritol dissolves. Add the ½ cup of melted coconut butter, vanilla and 2 teaspoons of rum. Let the mixture chill for 2 hours in the refrigerator.

3. Prepare the caramelized banana layer by sautéing the bananas in 1 tablespoon of coconut butter. Add 1 tablespoon of erythritol and cook until the bananas darken. Add the ¼ teaspoon of rum last. Adjust the heat to low and simmer for 5 minutes.

4. Assemble the dessert on a plate by layering the bananas and cooled cream, serve.

Nutrition:

Calories: 498

Carb: 30g

Protein: 7g

Deliciously Good Scones

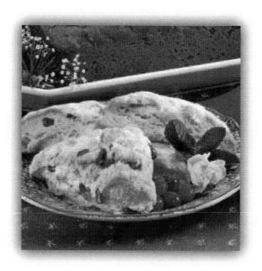

- ➤ Preparation time: 15 minutes
- ➤ Cooking time: 12 minutes
- ➤ Servings: 10
- ➤ Level of difficulty: Easy

Ingredients:

- ¼ cup dried apricots, chopped
- ¼ cup dried cranberries
- ¼ cup sunflower seeds
- ½ teaspoon baking soda
- 1 large egg
- 2 cups all-purpose flour
- 2 tablespoon honey

Directions:

1. Preheat the oven to 350F. Grease a baking sheet. Set aside. In a bowl, mix the salt, baking soda, and flour. Add the dried fruits, nuts, and seeds. Set aside.
2. In another bowl, mix the honey and eggs. Add the wet fixings to the dry ingredients. Use your hands to mix the dough.
3. Create 10 small round doughs and place them on the baking sheet—Bake for 12 minutes.

Nutrition:

Calories: 44

Carbs: 27g

Protein: 4g

Fats: 3g

Mixed Berry Cobbler

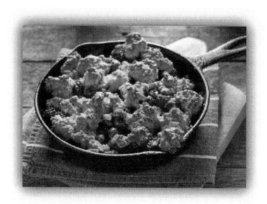

> Preparation time: 15 minutes
> Cooking time: 30 minutes
> Servings: 8
> Level of difficulty: Normal

Ingredients:

- ¼ cup of coconut milk
- ¼ cup ghee
- ¼ cup honey
- ½ cup almond flour
- ½ cup coconut flour
- ½ tablespoon cinnamon
- ½ tablespoon Erythtitol
- 1 teaspoon vanilla
- 12 ounces frozen raspberries
- 16 ounces frozen wild blueberries
- 2 teaspoon baking powder
- 2 teaspoon Arrow root

Directions:

1. Place the frozen berries in the slow cooker. Add honey and 2 teaspoons of Arrow root. Mix to combine.

2. In a bowl, mix the coconut four, almond flour, coconut milk, ghee, baking powder, and vanilla. Sweeten with Erythritol. Place this pastry mix on top of the berries. Set the oven to 350°F for 25 to 30 minutes.

Nutrition:

Calories: 146

Carbs: 33g

Protein: 1g

Fats: 6g

Blueberry Espresso Brownies

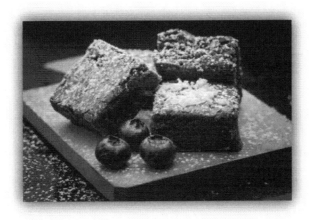

➢ Preparation time: 15 minutes
➢ Cooking time: 30 minutes
➢ Servings: 12
➢ Level of difficulty: Easy

Ingredients:

- ¼ cup organic cocoa powder
- ¼ teaspoon salt
- ½ cup raw honey
- ½ teaspoon baking soda

- 1 cup blueberries
- 1 cup coconut cream
- 1 tablespoon cinnamon
- 1 tablespoon ground coffee
- 2 teaspoon vanilla extract
- 3 eggs

Directions:

1. Preheat the oven to 3250F. In a bowl, mix coconut cream, honey, eggs, cinnamon, honey, vanilla, baking soda, coffee, and salt. Use a mixer to combine all ingredients. Fold in the blueberries
2. Put the batter in your greased baking dish, then bake for 30 minutes. Remove from the oven and let it cool.

Nutrition:

Calories: 168

Carbs: 20g

Protein: 4g

Fats: 10g

Coffee Brownies

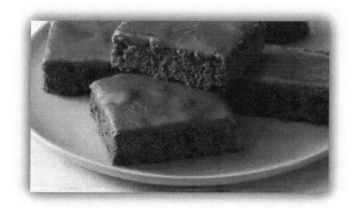

- ➢ Preparation time: 15 minutes
- ➢ Cooking time: 20 minutes
- ➢ Servings: 4
- ➢ Level of difficulty: Normal

Ingredients:

- 3 eggs, beaten
- 2 tablespoons cocoa powder
- 2 teaspoons Erythritol
- ½ cup almond flour
- ½ cup organic almond milk

Directions:

1. Put the eggs in your mixing bowl, then combine them with Erythritol and almond milk. With the help of the hand mixer, whisk the liquid until homogenous.
2. Then add almond flour and cocoa powder. Whisk the mixture until smooth. Take the non-sticky brownie mold and transfer the cocoa mass inside it.
3. Flatten it using a spatula. The flattened mass should be thin—Preheat the oven to 365F. Transfer the brownie to the oven and bake it for 20 minutes.
4. Then chill the cooked brownies at least till room temperature and cut into serving bars.

Nutrition:

Calories 78

Fat 5.8g

Carbs 2.7g

Protein 5.5g

Fragrant Lava Cake

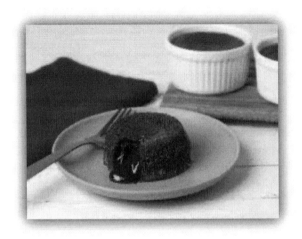

- ➢ Preparation time: 10 minutes
- ➢ Cooking time: 15 minutes
- ➢ Servings: 5
- ➢ Level of difficulty: Normal

Ingredients:

- 1 teaspoon baking powder
- 1 teaspoon vanilla extract
- 2 eggs, whisked
- 4 tablespoons cocoa powder
- 2 tablespoons Erythritol
- 8 tablespoons heavy cream
- 4 teaspoon almond flour

- Butter for greasing

Directions:

1. Whisk the eggs together with heavy cream. Then add vanilla extract, Erythritol, cocoa powder, and almond flour. Mix the mixture until smooth.

2. Spray the mini cake molds with the butter. Preheat the oven to 350F. Pour the cake mixture into the cake molds and place in the oven.

3. Bake the cakes for 15 minutes. Then remove the lava cakes from the oven and discard them from the cake molds. Serve the lava cakes only hot.

Nutrition:

Calories 218

Fat 19.1g

Carbs 8.3g

Protein 8.1g

Almond Butter Mousse

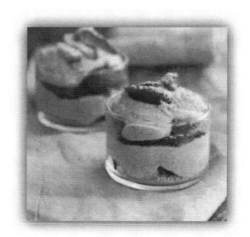

- ➤ Preparation time: 7 minutes
- ➤ Cooking time: 7 minutes
- ➤ Servings: 3
- ➤ Level of difficulty: Easy

Ingredients:

- 2 strawberries
- 1 cup of coconut milk
- ½ teaspoon vanilla extract
- 2 teaspoon Erythritol
- 4 tablespoons almond butter
- ¾ teaspoon ground cinnamon

Directions:

1. Pour coconut milk into the food processor. Add vanilla extract, Erythritol, almond butter, and ground cinnamon. Blend the mixture until smooth.
2. Then transfer it in the saucepan and start to preheat it over medium heat. Stir it all the time. When the mousse begins to be thick, remove it from the heat and stir.
3. Allow to cool. Pour mousse into serving glasses.
4. Slice the strawberries, and layer them in the mousse. Decorate with almond granules and serve.

Nutrition:

Calories 321

Fat 31.1g

Carbs 9.6g

Protein 6.4g

Smoothie and Healthy Drinks

Winter Berry Smoothie

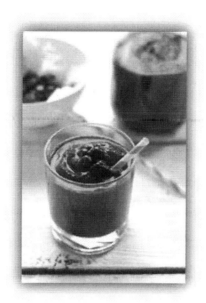

- ➤ Preparation Time: 5 minutes
- ➤ Servings: 2
- ➤ Level of difficulty: Easy

Ingredients:

- 1/4 cup blackberries
- 1/4 cup cherries, pitted
- 1/4 cup cranberries
- 2 cups of water

Directions:

1. Blend until smooth in a blender or smoothie maker. Serve right away.

Nutrition:

Calories: 21

Fat: 0 g

Carbs: 5 g

Protein: 2 g

Carrot Smoothie

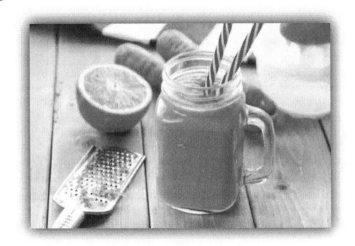

> ➢ Preparation Time: 5 minutes
> ➢ Servings: 1
> ➢ Level of difficulty: Easy

Ingredients:

- 1 cup cut carrots

- ½ teaspoon finely destroyed an orange strip

- 1 cup squeezed orange

- 1½ cups of ice 3D shapes

- Orange strip twists (to decorate)

Directions:

1. In a secured little pan, cook carrots in a modest quantity of bubbling water for around 15 minutes or until delicate. Channel well. Cool.

2. Spot depleted carrots in a blender. Include finely destroyed orange strip and squeezed orange. Cover and mix until smooth.

3. Put the ice blocks; cover and mix until smooth. Fill glasses. Whenever wanted, decorate with orange strip twists.

Nutrition:

Calories: 97

Fat: 0.6 g

Carbs: 22.4 g

Protein: 0 g

Strawberry Papaya Smoothie

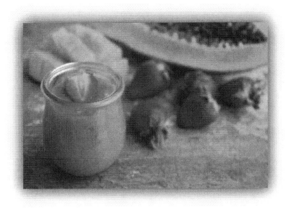

➤ Preparation Time: 10 minutes

➤ Servings: 1

➤ Level of difficulty: Easy

Ingredients:

- ½ cup of strawberries
- 2 cups of sliced papaya
- 2 cup of coconut kefir
- 2 scoop of vanilla bone-broth protein powder
- ½ cup of ice water

Directions:

1. Add all the above fixings to the blender & blend on high until smooth. Serve.

Nutrition:

Calories: 196.9

Fat: 1.5 g

Carbs: 28 g

Protein: 19.6 g

Gut Cleansing Smoothie

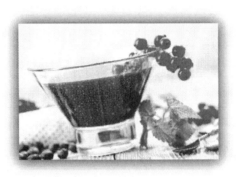

➤ Preparation Time: 10 minutes
➤ Servings: 1
➤ Level of difficulty: Easy

Ingredients:

- 1 ½ tablespoons coconut oil, unrefined
- ½ cup plain full-fat yogurt
- 1 tablespoon chia seeds
- 1 serving aloe Vera leaves
- ½ cup frozen blueberries, unsweetened
- 1 tablespoon hemp hearts
- 1 cup of water
- 1 scoop Pinnaclife prebiotic fiber

Directions:

1. Blend all listed ingredients to a blender until you have a smooth plus creamy texture. Serve chilled and enjoy!

Nutrition:

Calories: 298

Fat: 33 g

Carbs: 8 g

Protein: 12 g

Cabbage and Chia Glass

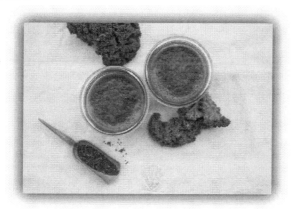

> ➢ Preparation Time: 10 minutes
> ➢ Servings: 2
> ➢ Level of difficulty: Easy

Ingredients:

- 1/3 cup cabbage
- 1 cup cold unsweetened almond milk
- 1 tablespoon chia seeds
- ½ lemon juice
- ½ cup lettuce

Directions:

1. Add coconut milk to your blender. Cut cabbage and add to your blender. Put the chia seeds in your coffee grinder and chop to powder; brush the powder into a blender.

2. Wash and dry the lettuce and chop. Add to the mix, whit the lemon juice, cover and blend on low, followed by the medium. Taste the texture and serve chilled!

Nutrition:

Calories: 209

Fat: 23 g

Carbs: 8 g

Protein: 12 g

Almonds and Zucchini Smoothie

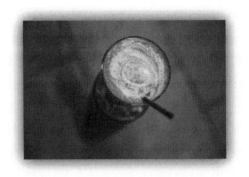

- ➢ Preparation Time: 5 minutes
- ➢ Servings: 2
- ➢ Level of difficulty: Easy

Ingredients:

- 1 cup zucchini, cooked and mashed - unsalted
- 1 1/2 cups almond milk
- 1 tbsp almond butter (plain, unsalted)
- 1 tsp pure almond extract
- 2 tbsp ground almonds or Macadamia almonds
- 1/2 cup water
- 1 cup Ice cubes crushed (optional, for serving)

Directions:

1. Dump all fixings from the list above in your fast-speed blender; blend for 45 - 60 seconds or taste. Serve with crushed ice.

Nutrition:

Calories: 322

Fat: 30 g

Carbs: 6 g

Protein: 6 g

Baby Spinach and Dill Smoothie

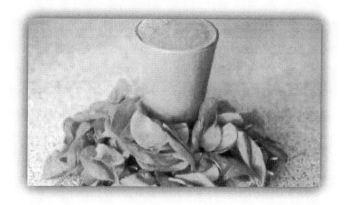

➤ Preparation Time: 5 minutes
➤ Servings: 2
➤ Level of difficulty: Easy

Ingredients:

- 1 cup of fresh baby spinach leaves
- 2 tbsp of fresh dill, chopped
- 1 1/2 cup of water
- 1/2 avocado, chopped into cubes
- 1 tbsp chia seeds (optional)

- 2 tbsp of natural sweetener Stevia or Erythritol (optional)

Directions:

1. Place all fixings into a fast-speed blender. Beat until smooth and all Ingredients united well. Serve and enjoy!

Nutrition:

Calories: 136

Fat: 10 g

Carbs: 8 g

Protein: 7 g

Blueberries and Coconut Smoothie

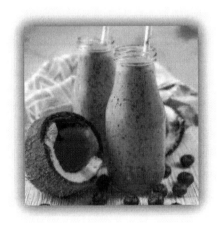

- ➢ Preparation Time: 5 minutes
- ➢ Servings: 5
- ➢ Level of difficulty: Easy

Ingredients:

- 1 cup of frozen blueberries, unsweetened
- 1 cup Stevia or Erythritol sweetener
- 2 cups of coconut milk (canned)
- 1 cup of fresh spinach leaves

- 2 tbsp shredded coconut (unsweetened)
- 3/4 cup water

Directions:

1. Place all fixings from the list in the food processor or your strong blender. Blend for 45 - 60 seconds or to taste. Ready for a drink! Serve!

Nutrition:

Calories: 190

Fat: 18 g

Carbs: 8 g

Protein: 3 g

Apple-Cinnamon Drink

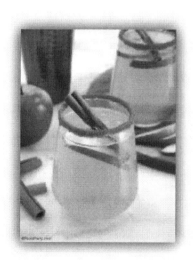

- ➢ Preparation time: 10 minutes
- ➢ Servings: 8
- ➢ Level of difficulty: Easy

Ingredients:

- 10 cups water

- 1 medium apple, sliced
- 2 cinnamon sticks
- 2 teaspoons ground cinnamon

Directions:

1. Add apple slices, water, and cinnamon to a blender. Pour this mixture along with cinnamon stick into a suitable cooking pot and cook for 5 minutes. Strain the apple cinnamon water and allow it to cool. Serve.

Nutrition:

Calories: 4

Fat: 0 g

Carbs: 1 g

Protein: 0 g

Blackberry-Sage Drink

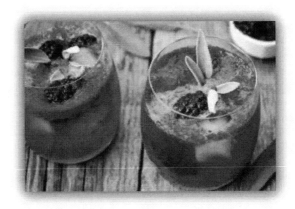

- ➢ Preparation time: 10 minutes
- ➢ Servings: 8
- ➢ Level of difficulty: Easy

Ingredients:

- 1 cup fresh blackberries

- 4 sage leaves

- 10 cups water

Directions:

1. Add blackberries, sage leave, and 10 cups water to a blender. Blend well, then strain and refrigerate to chill. Serve.

Nutrition:

Calories: 7

Fat: 0 g

Carbs: 2 g

Protein: 0 g

Apple Beet Juice Blend

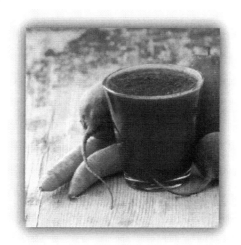

➤ Preparation time: 10 minutes
➤ Servings: 2
➤ Level of difficulty: Easy

Ingredients:

- ½ medium apple
- ½ medium beet

- 1 medium fresh carrot
- 1 celery stalk
- ¼ cup parsley

Directions:

1. Put the apple, beet, celery, parsley, and carrot through a juicer. Divide this juice into two serving glasses, then refrigerate to chill. Serve.

Nutrition:

Calories: 186

Fat: 2 g

Carbs: 19 g

Protein: 23 g

Caramel Protein Latte

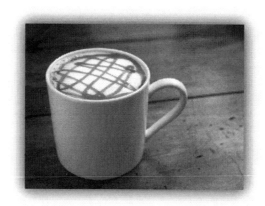

➤ Preparation time: 10 minutes
➤ Servings: 2
➤ Level of difficulty: Easy

Ingredients:

- 1 scoop whey protein powder

- 2 ounces of water
- 6 ounces hot coffee
- 2 tablespoons caramel syrup

Directions:

1. Mix 1 scoop of protein powder with 2 ounces of water in a mug. Pour in 6 ounces of hot coffee, then mix well. Stir in sugar-free syrup and serve.

Nutrition:

Calories: 72

Fat: 0 g

Carbs: 1 g

Protein: 17 g

Cinnamon Smoothie

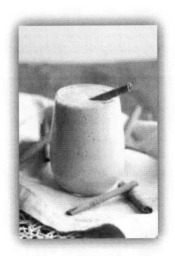

➤ Preparation time: 10 minutes
➤ Servings: 2
➤ Level of difficulty: Easy

Ingredients:

- ½ teaspoon ground cinnamon
- 1 tablespoon sugar
- 1/8 teaspoon vanilla extract
- 8 ounces egg white
- 3 tablespoons whipped unsweetened cream

Directions:

1. Mix cinnamon, sugar, 2 ounces egg whites, and vanilla in a mixer. Serve with whipped topping. Enjoy.

Nutrition:

Calories: 207

Fat: 3 g

Carbs: 17 g

Protein: 28 g

Raspberry and Pineapple Smoothie

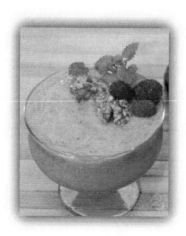

➤ Preparation Time: 5 minutes
➤ Servings: 4

➤ Level of difficulty: Easy

Ingredients:

- 1 chopped small overripe banana piece
- 8 oz. rinsed and drained pineapple tidbits
- ½ cup frozen raspberries
- ½ cup crushed ice

Directions:

1. Blend all fruit in a high speed blender. Pour into 4 large glasses, decorate with walnuts or cashews, a mint leaf, and enjoy cold.

Nutrition:

Calories: 360

Fat: 1 g

Carbs: 90 g

Protein: 3.1 g

Power-Boosting Smoothie

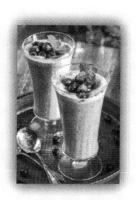

➤ Preparation Time: 5 minutes
➤ Servings: 2
➤ Level of difficulty: Easy

Ingredients:

- ½ cup of water
- ½ cup non-dairy whipped topping
- 2 scoops whey protein powder
- 1½ cups frozen blueberries

Directions:

1. In a high-speed blender, add all fixings and pulse till smooth. Transfer into 2 serving glass and serve immediately.

Nutrition:

Calories: 242

Fat: 7 g

Carbs: 23.8 g

Protein: 23.2 g

Digestive Smoothie

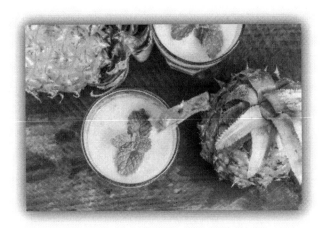

- ➤ Preparation Time: 5 minutes
- ➤ Servings: 2
- ➤ Level of difficulty: Easy

Ingredients:

- ¼ cup crushed ice cubes
- 2 scoops of vanilla whey protein powder
- 1 cup of water
- 1½ cups pineapple

Directions:

1. In a high-speed blender, add all fixings and pulse till smooth. Transfer into 2 serving glass and serve immediately.

Nutrition:

Calories: 117

Fat: 2.1 g

Carbs: 18.2 g

Protein: 22.7 g

Strengthening Smoothie Bowl

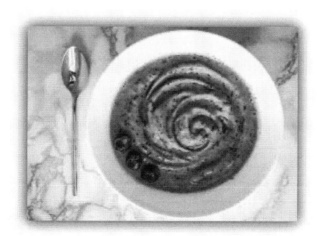

- ➢ Preparation Time: 5 minutes
- ➢ Servings: 2
- ➢ Level of difficulty: Easy

Ingredients:

- ¼ cup fresh or frozen blueberries
- ¼ cup fat-free plain Greek yogurt
- 1/3 cup unsweetened almond milk
- 2 tbsps whey protein powder
- 2 tbsp fresh blueberries

Directions:

2. In a blender, add frozen blueberries and pulse for about 1 minute. Add almond milk, yogurt, and protein powder and pulse till desired consistency.
3. Transfer the mixture into 2 bowls evenly. Serve with the topping of fresh blueberries.

Nutrition:

Calories: 176

Fat: 2.1 g

Carbs: 27 g

Protein: 15.1 g

Antioxidant Berry Smoothie

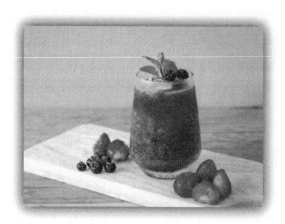

- ➤ Preparation Time: 5 minutes
- ➤ Servings: 2

➤ Level of difficulty: Easy

Ingredients:

- ¼ cup blackberries
- ¼ cup of unenriched rice milk.
- ¼ cup sliced strawberries
- ¼ cup blueberries

Directions:

1. Blend in using a food processor or smoothie maker and serve over ice if desired. Enjoy!

Nutrition:

Calories: 90

Fat: 1 g

Carbs: 18 g

Protein: 1 g

Berry and Almond Smoothie

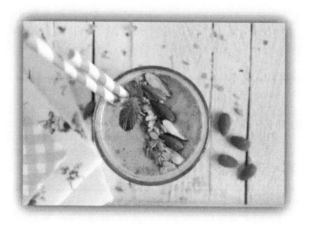

- ➢ Preparation Time: 10 minutes
- ➢ Servings: 4
- ➢ Level of difficulty: Easy

Ingredients:

- 1 cup of blueberries, frozen
- 1 whole banana
- ½ a cup of almond milk
- 1 tablespoon of almond butter
- Chopped almonds
- Water as needed

Directions:

1. Add the listed ingredients to your blender and blend well until you have a smoothie-like texture. Decorate whit chopped almonds and serve. Enjoy!

Nutrition:

Calories: 321

Fat: 11 g

Carbs: 55 g

Protein: 5 g

Mango and Pear Smoothie

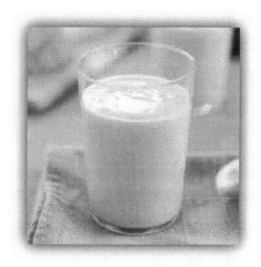

- ➢ Preparation Time: 10 minutes
- ➢ Servings: 1
- ➢ Level of difficulty: Easy

Ingredients:

- 1 ripe mango, cored and chopped
- ½ mango, peeled, pitted, and chopped
- 1 cup kale, chopped
- ½ cup plain Greek yogurt
- 2 ice cubes

Directions:

1. Add pear, mango, yogurt, kale, and mango to a blender and puree. Put ice, then blend until you have a smooth texture. Serve and enjoy!

Nutrition:

Calories: 193

Fat: 8 g

Carbs: 53 g rotein: 8 g

Keto Coffee Smoothie

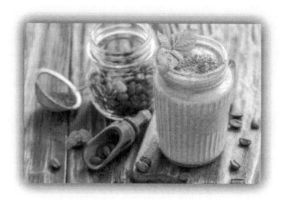

- ➤ Preparation time: 10 minutes
- ➤ Servings: 1
- ➤ Level of difficulty: Easy

Ingredients:

- 2 cups strongly brewed coffee, chilled
- ½ cup water
- 1-ounce Macadamia nuts
- 1 tablespoon chia seeds
- ½ teaspoon raw cocoa powder
- 1 pinch cinnamon
- 1-2 teaspoons Stevia, optional
- 1 tablespoon MCT oil

Directions:

1. Grind chia seeds and macadamia nuts in a coffee grinder until reduced to a powder.
2. Add all the listed fixings to a blender. Blend on high until smooth and creamy. Enjoy your smoothie.

Nutrition:

Calories: 325

Fat: 39g

Carbohydrates: 11g

Protein: 5.2g

Blackberry and Apple Smoothie

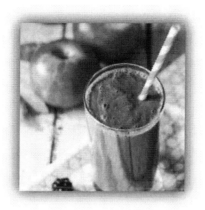

- ➢ Preparation time: 5 minutes
- ➢ Servings: 2
- ➢ Level of difficulty: Easy

Ingredients:

- 1 cup frozen blackberries
- ½ cup apple cider
- 1 apple, cubed
- 2/3 cup non-fat lemon yogurt

Directions:

1. Add the listed ingredients to your blender and blend until smooth. Serve chilled!

Nutrition:

Calories: 200

Fat: 10g

Carbohydrates: 14g

Protein 2g

Minty Cherry Smoothie

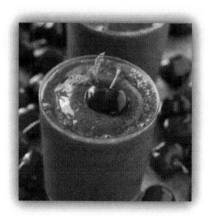

- ➢ Preparation time: 5 minutes
- ➢ Servings: 2
- ➢ Level of difficulty: Easy

Ingredients:

- ¾ cup cherries, sliced, pitted
- 1 teaspoon mint
- ½ cup almond milk
- ½ cup kale
- ½ teaspoon fresh vanilla

Directions:

1. Add cherries to the blender, then pour almond milk. Wash the mint and put two sprigs in the blender. Separate the kale leaves from the stems
2. Put kale in a blender. Press vanilla bean and cut lengthwise with a knife. Scoop out your desired amount of vanilla and add to the blender. Blend until smooth. Serve chilled and enjoy!

Nutrition:

Calories: 200

Fat: 10g

Carbohydrates: 14g

Protein 2g

Vitaminic Coconut Smoothie

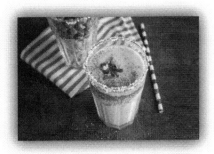

➢ Preparation time: 10 minutes
➢ Servings: 1
➢ Level of difficulty: Easy

Ingredients:

- 1 cup of coconut milk
- 1 cup of water
- tablespoons of blueberries
- 1 teaspoon stevia, optional
- 1 tablespoon coconut flakes
- tablespoons pecans, chopped
- 1 tablespoon chopped almonds

Directions:

1. Pour the coconut milk, flakes, water, and nuts into a blender. Blend on high speed until mixture is smooth and creamy. Pour into a large glass and add the blueberries and chia seeds and let stand 10 minutes. Create a topping with the chopped nuts and coconut flakes. Taste.1 cup of spring mix salad blend

Nutrition:

Calories: 385

Fat: 34g

Carbohydrates: 16g

Protein: 6.9g

Green Minty Smoothie

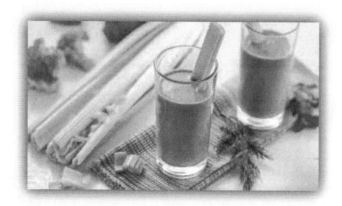

- ➤ Preparation time: 10 minutes
- ➤ Servings: 1
- ➤ Level of difficulty: Easy

Ingredients:

- 1 stalk celery
- 2 cups of water
- 2 ounces almonds
- 1 teaspoon Erythritol
- 2 mint leaves

Directions:

1. Add listed ingredients to a blender. Blend until you have a smooth plus creamy texture. Serve chilled and enjoy!

Nutrition:

Calories: 287

Fat: 25g

Carbohydrates: 13g

Protein: 5.5g

Salad Recipes

Pear & Brie Salad

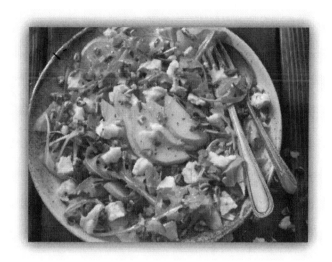

- ➢ Preparation time: 5 minutes
- ➢ Servings: 4
- ➢ Level of difficulty: Easy

Ingredients:

- 1 cup arugula
- ¼ cup chopped brie
- ½ lemon
- ½ cup fresh pears, diced
- 1 tbsp. olive oil
- ¼ cup crumbled walnuts

Directions:

1. Wash the arugula and arrange in a serving bowl with the sliced pears.
2. Crumble the brie and walnuts on top. Whisk the olive oil and lemon juice together.
3. Season with a little black pepper to taste and serve immediately.

Nutrition:

Calories 54

Protein 1 g

Carbs 12 g

Fat 7 g

Caesar Salad

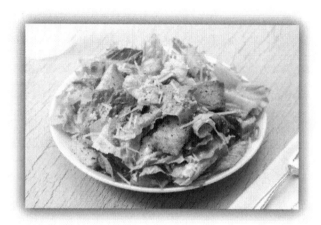

- ➤ Preparation time: 5 minutes
- ➤ Servings: 4
- ➤ Level of difficulty: Easy

Ingredients:

- 1 head romaine lettuce
- ¼ cup mayonnaise
- 4 tbsps. Parmesan cheese flakes
- 1 tbsp. lemon juice
- 8 anchovy fillets
- 1 tsp. Worcestershire sauce
- 1 cup of roasted stale bread pieces
- Black pepper
- 1 garlic cloves
- 1 tsp. mustard

Directions:

1. In a small bowl combine the mayonnaise, mustard, minced garlic clove, and lemon juice and whisk with a fork.
2. Cut up the lettuce and place on serving plates, pour over the prepared dressing, add the anchovy fillets, Parmesan cheese and toasted stale bread pieces while still warm.

Nutrition:

Calories 44

Fat 2.1 g

Carbs 4.3 g

Protein 3.2 g

Cucumber and Red Onion Salad

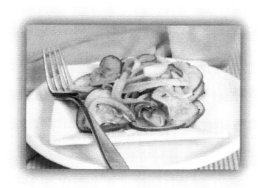

➢ Preparation time: 5 minutes
➢ Servings: 4
➢ Level of difficulty: Easy

Ingredients:

- 3 cucumbers
- 1 tbsp. dried dill
- 1 red onion
- ¼ cup of water

- 1 tbsp extra virgin olive oil
- 1 cup apple cider vinegar
- 2 tbsps brown sugar

Directions:

1. Peel the cucumbers and onion, and thinly slice them.
2. Create a vinaigrette with the apple cider vinegar, oil, water, brown sugar and dill.
3. In a bowl, add all the ingredients, stir, and allow 20 to 30 minutes to marinate in the dressing. Serve.

Nutrition:

Calories 49

Fat 0.1g

Protein 0.8g

Carbs 11g

Thai Cucumber and peanut Salad

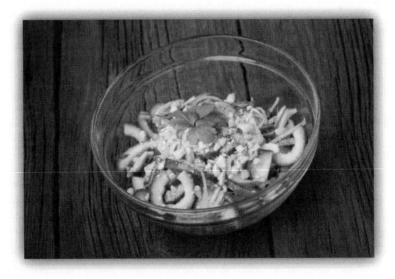

➢ Preparation time: 5 minutes
➢ Servings: 2
➢ Level of difficulty: Easy

Ingredients:

- 2 cucumbers
- ½ red onion
- ¼ cup chopped peanuts
- ¼ cup brown sugar
- ½ cup cilantro
- ¼ cup rice wine vinegar
- 2 jalapeno peppers

Directions:

1. Wash the cucumbers and remove the inside of the seeds. Cut them into slices. Slice the onion.
2. Prepare a vinaigrette with vinegar, sugar and oil.
3. In a bowl, add all components and mix well. Serve with dressing.

Nutrition:

Calories 20

Fat 0g

Carbs 5g

Protein 1g

Healthy Potato Salad

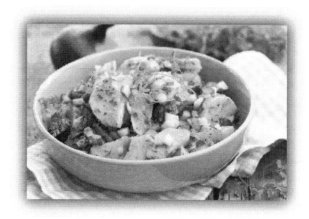

> ➤ Preparation time: 5 minutes
> ➤ Cooking time: 10 minutes
> ➤ Servings: 2
> ➤ Level of difficulty: Easy

Ingredients:

- 300 gr of potatoes
- ½ fresh zucchini in chunks
- 1 red onion, chopped
- 1 tablespoon fresh walnuts
- 1 tablespoon apple vinegar
- 1 pinch of salt
- 1 bunch of parsley
- 1 garlic clove
- 1 squeezed lemon
- ½ cup extra virgin olive oil
- Pepper

Directions:

1. Peel the potatoes and cut them into chunks. Steam them for 15 minutes or until tender.

2. Meanwhile, create an emulsion by chopping the parsley, garlic, and juice of one squeezed lemon with an immersion blender.2 cups mayonnaise

3. Take the warmed potatoes, pour them into a large bowl, and combine all the ingredients. Season with the emulsion and pepper and enjoy.

Nutrition:

Calories 280

Fat 20 g

Carbs 26 g

Protein 2 g

Broccoli-Cauliflower Salad

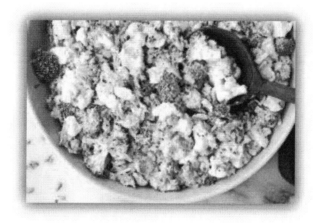

➢ Preparation time: 5 minutes

➢ Cooking time: 10 minutes

➢ Servings: 4

➢ Level of difficulty: Easy

Ingredients:

- 1 cup cauliflower florets
- 2 tpsps brown sugar
- 4 hard-cooked eggs
- 5 slices bacon
- 1 cup broccoli florets

- 1 cup organic whipping sugar-free cream
- 1 tbsp. wine apple vinegar

Directions:

1. Steam the broccoli and cauliflower for 10 minutes (they should remain crispy). Cool and set aside.
2. Using a whisk, beat the cream, apple cider vinegar, and brown sugar to create a sauce.
3. Cut hard-boiled eggs into small pieces and combine with bacon.
4. In a large bowl, combine all the elements and mix well. Serve with the dressing.

Nutrition:

Calories 89.8

Fat 4.5 g

Carbs 11.5 g

Protein 3.0 g

Grilled Turkey Salad

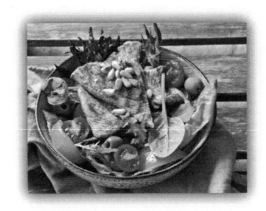

- ➢ Preparation time: 10 minutes
- ➢ Cooking time: 6 minutes
- ➢ Servings: 2
- ➢ Level of difficulty: Easy

Ingredients:

- 220 gr of turkey breast
- ½ cup of pitted green olives
- 1 cup cherry tomatoes
- 250 gr of mixed field salad
- 1 bell pepper cut into fillets and seeds removed
- 2 tablespoons lemon juice
- 2 tablespoons olive oil
- 2 tablespoons pine nuts

Directions:

1. Heat a griddle and when hot, place turkey slices on it, about 3 minutes per side, or until well cooked and browned.
2. In a saucepan of boiling water, pour the bell pepper fillets and blanch for 5 minutes, drain and run under cold water. Peel them if possible.
3. In a small pan, toast the pine nuts and set aside.
4. Wash the mixed field salad, dry it and arrange it on 2 serving plates, with the coarsely chopped turkey slices, the peppers, the cherry tomatoes, the olives and lastly the pine nuts.
5. Dress with oil and lemon, and serve.

Nutrition:

Calories 260

Fat 11 g

Carbs 16 g

Protein 20 g

Green Bean and Potato Salad

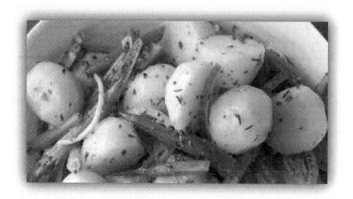

- ➤ Preparation time: 5 minutes
- ➤ Cooking time: 25 minutes
- ➤ Servings: 4
- ➤ Level of difficulty: Easy

Ingredients:

- 1 lb. red potatoes
- ¾ lb. green beans
- ½ cup basil
- ¼ cup olive oil
- 1 tbsp. mustard
- 1 tbsp. lemon juice
- ½ cup balsamic vinegar
- 1 red onion
- 1 garlic clove

Directions:

1. Put the potatoes in your pot with water, then boil for 15-18 minutes or until tender. Thrown in green beans after 5-6 minutes. Drain and cut into cubes.
2. Mince the garlic and chop the onion.
3. In a bowl, create an emulsion with mustard, lemon juice, olive oil, and balsamic vinegar.
4. Combine all ingredients and mix well. Serve with the dressing.

Nutrition:

Calories 153.2

Fat 2 g

Carbs 29 g

Protein 6.9 g

Beet and Cucumber Salad

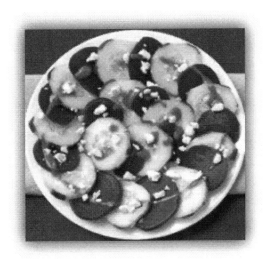

> ➢ Preparation Time: 10 minutes
> ➢ Servings: 6
> ➢ Level of difficulty: Easy

Ingredients:

- 1 cucumber, thinly sliced
- 15 ounces of canned low sodium sliced beets
- 4 teaspoons of balsamic vinegar
- 2 teaspoons of olive oil
- 2 tablespoons of Feta cheese

Directions:

1. Place the slices of beet on a serving plate. Layer the slices of cucumber over the beet slices. Drizzle layered beet slices with vinegar and oil. Sprinkle drizzled beet slices with crumbled Feta cheese.

Nutrition:

Calories 74

Protein 1g

Carbohydrates 13g

Fat 2g

Chicken Apple Crunch Salad

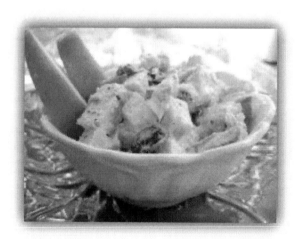

- ➢ Preparation Time: 30 minutes
- ➢ Cooking Time: 0 minutes
- ➢ Servings: 4
- ➢ Level of difficulty: Easy

Ingredients:

- • 2 cups of cooked chicken
- • 2 green apples

- 2 tablespoons of scallions
- ¼ cup of dark raisins
- 1/3 cup of low-fat mayonnaise
- 1 tablespoon of low-fat sour cream
- 1 teaspoon of lemon juice
- ¼ teaspoon of cinnamon
- ¼ teaspoon of black pepper

Directions:

1. Cook the chicken in a thick-bottomed skillet, basting occasionally with water to avoid browning. Continue cooking for 15 minutes or until the chicken is soft and fully cooked.

2. Cube the cooked chicken, dice the apple and celery, and chop the scallions. Use a large salad bowl to combine and mix the chicken, apple, celery, scallions, and raisins.

3. Whisk together the mayonnaise, lemon juice, sour cream, cinnamon, and black pepper.

4. Pour on top of the chicken apple mixture and toss. Put in the fridge to chill before serving.

Nutrition:

Calories 244

Protein 21g

Carbohydrates 13g

Fat 12g

Grilled Peach, Arugula and Ricotta Cheese Salad

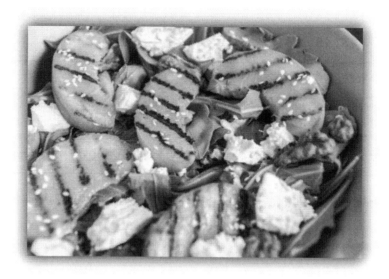

- ➢ Preparation Time: 10 minutes
- ➢ Cooking Time: 5 minutes
- ➢ Servings: 2
- ➢ Level of difficulty: Easy

Ingredients:

- 300 gr of arugula
- 2 medium peaches, not too ripe
- 250 gr of fresh sheep ricotta
- 4 walnuts
- 1 tablespoon of extra virgin olive oil
- 1 tablespoon maple syrup
- 1 pinch of salt

Directions:

1. Wash the arugula and dry it well. Crack the walnuts and set the kernels aside.
2. Peel the peaches, cut them into slices and grill them on a griddle for 5 minutes, turning once on each side.
3. Compose the dish with the arugula, peaches, walnuts, a pinch of salt, oil and maple syrup.

Nutrition:

Calories 81

Protein 10 g

Carb. 10 g

Fats 13 g

Fruited Curry Chicken Salad

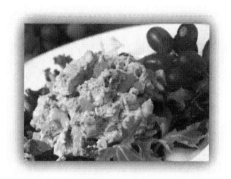

➢ Preparation Time: 45 minutes

➢ Servings: 2

➢ Level of difficulty: Normal

Ingredients:

- 1 cooked skinless and boneless chicken breasts
- 1 stalk of celery
- ½ cup of onion
- 1 medium-sized apple
- ¼ cup of seedless red grapes
- ½ cup of dried apricots
- 1/8 teaspoon of black pepper
- ½ teaspoon of curry powder
- ¾ cup of homade mayonnaise

Directions:

1. Dice the chicken and chop the celery, onion, apricots, and apple.

2. Mix the chicken, celery, apple, grapes, onion, apricots, pepper, curry powder, and mayonnaise in a large bowl. Toss all ingredients together, then serve or chill for later.

Nutrition:

Calories 238   Fat 18g

Protein 14g   Carbohydrates 6g

Powerful Salad

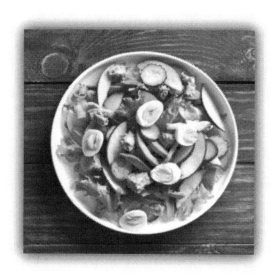

- ➤ Preparation Time: 10 minutes
- ➤ Cooking Time: 10 minutes
- ➤ Servings: 2
- ➤ Level of difficulty: Easy

Ingredients:

- 250 gr of drained tuna fillets
- 2 eggs
- 300 gr field salad
- 1 apple of medium size

- 1 cucumber
- 1 tablespoon of apple vinegar

Directions:

1. Put the eggs in some water and hard-boil them. Cool them under running water.
2. Wash and dry the salad. Slice the cucumber.
3. In a large dish, place the salad, tuna, hard-boiled eggs cut in two, apple slices, cucumber slices, season with apple cider vinegar.

Nutrition:

Calories 157

Protein 30 g

Carbohydrates 24 g

Fat 21 g

Greek Style Chickpea Pasta Salad

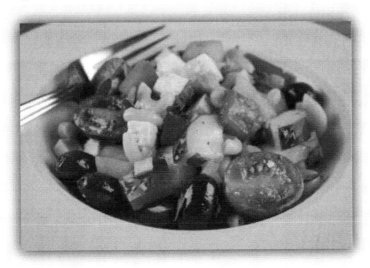

- ➢ Preparation Time: 20 minutes
- ➢ Cooking Time: 10 minutes

- ➢ Servings: 4
- ➢ Level of difficulty: Normal

Ingredients:

- 250 gr of chickpea pasta
- 1 ½ cup of cherry tomatoes cut in half
- ½ cup of Cammarata olives
- 125 gr feta cheese
- tablespoons dijon mustard
- 1 tablespoon maple syrup
- 1 cucumber
- 1 red bell bell pepper
- 1 bunch of basil
- tablespoons of extra virgin olive oil
- 1 pinch of salt

Directions:

1. Cook the chickpea pasta in boiling salted water and drain when al dente. Leave to cool under running water.
2. Prepare a dressing by combining the extra virgin olive oil, mustard, maple syrup and a pinch of salt. Whisk with a fork until the liquids are combined.
3. Cut the bell bell pepper into strips and the cucumber into chunks.
4. Cut the feta into small squares.
5. In a large bowl pour all the ingredients, and dress with the hand-prepared sauce. Serve or keep refrigerated and let cool further.

Nutrition:

Calories 260

Protein 16 g

Carbohydrates 18 g

Fat 14g

Spinach-Mandarin Salad

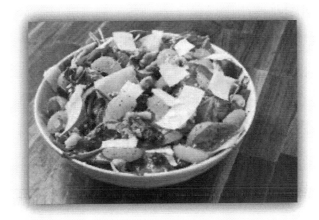

- ➤ Preparation Time: 20 minutes
- ➤ Servings: 2
- ➤ Level of difficulty: Easy

Ingredients:

- 2 cups of fresh spinach
- ½ cup dried cranberries
- 1 cup tangerines, skinned
- 1 medium-sized apple, cut into wedges
- ½ cup parmesan flakes
- ¼ cup walnut kernels
- tablespoons rice or apple vinegar
- tablespoons olive oil
- ½ lemon, squeezed
- 1 pinch black pepper
- 1 pinch of salt

Directions:

1. In a large bowl place the washed and drained spinach, sprinkle with the dried blueberries. Add the apple segments, tangerines and walnuts.

2. Prepare the vinaigrette with the oil, vinegar, salt, lemon, and pepper and whisk well with a fork.

3. Dress the salad with the vinaigrette and sprinkle with Parmesan flakes.

Nutrition:

Calories 117

Protein 2g

Carbohydrates 21g

Fat 4g

The 28-Days Meal Plan & Shopping List

Shopping List Week 1

Kamut flour, rice flour, almond butter, almond milk, aloe Vera leaves, apple cider vinegar, avocado, peas, blackberries, blueberries, bread crumbs, broccoli, brown rice, brown sugar, barley, bulgur, butter, kale, cumin seeds, carrots, cauliflower, celery, lentils, cherries, chia seeds, chicken, chicken broth, chili powder, cilantro, cinnamon, coconut kefir, coconut butter, corn, cornmeal, cornstarch, blueberries, light cream cheese, cucumbers, Dijon mustard, dried parsley, dried thyme, dried lentils, eggs, eggplant, extra virgin olive oil, fennel, unsalted bread, whole wheat flour, tortillas, fresh spinach leaves, fresh dill, garlic, Granny Smith apple, green peppers, green chilies, ground almonds, Macadamia nuts, ground beef, ground black pepper, ground cumin, ground nutmeg, sugar-free organic whipping cream, hemp seeds, dry herb seasoning mix, honey, kale, lemon, lettuce, sweet potato, ghee, parsley, lime, lettuce leaves, low-fat vanilla yogurt, canned low-sodium tuna in water, low-fat mayonnaise, low-fat milk, maple syrup, mint leaves, mustard seeds, natural sweetener Stevia, erythritol, onion, oranges, barley, papaya, paprika, white wine, parmesan cheese, Brussels sprouts, sun-dried tomatoes, green olives, radishes, arugula, apple cider vinegar, plain whole yogurt, pork chops, pumpkin, red apple, red cabbage, red onion, red peppers, roast beef, Roma tomatoes, salt, shallots, sirloin steak, skim milk, phosphate-free baking powder, sour cream, soy sauce, strawberries, sweet bell pepper, sweet potatoes, tomato sauce, turmeric, unsalted pasture butter, unsweetened apple mousse, vanilla protein powder, vanilla extract, wheat bran, white onion, white rice, brown sugar, whole wheat bread, whole wheat flour, golden onion, Pinnaclife prebiotic fiber, low-fat natural yogurt, zucchinis.

Meal Plan Week 1

Day	Breakfast	Lunch	Dinner	Snacks/Sides	Smoothies/Drinks
1	Breakfast Salad from Grains & Fruits	Roast beef wraps	Veal meatloaf with herbs	Cabbage Apple Stir-Fry	Winter Berry Smoothie
2	French Toast with Applesauce	Beef flans	Tuna and asparagus salad	Parmesan Roasted Cauliflower	Carrot Smoothie
3	Bagels made Healthy	Beef Burritos	Chicken salad	Celery and Fennel Salad with Cranberries	Strawberry Papaya Smoothie
4	Cornbread with Southern Twist	Pork chops with pesto	Stir-fried broccoli and beef	Kale with Caramelized Onions	Gut Cleansing Smoothie
5	Grandma's Pancake Special	Rice cakes	Eggplant meatballs	Italian Peas and Mint Risotto	Cabbage and Chia Glass
6	Pasta with Indian Lentils	Roasted bread with creamy mustard eggs	Green pepper fillet	Spicy Baked Sweet Potato Wedges	Almonds and Zucchini Smoothie
7	Apple Pumpkin Muffins	Stuffed peppers	Cucumber cream	Delicious veggies in apple cider vinegar	Baby Spinach and Dill Smoothie

Shopping List Week 2

Almond milk, apple, asparagus, baking powder, banana, bay leaf, beet, blackberries, blueberries, butter, caramel, carrots, Konjac noodles, pine nuts, broccoli, anchovies, pecorino romano, cauliflower, cayenne pepper, celery stalk, chickpeas, chili powder, chives, cilantro, cinnamon sticks, coconut milk, corn, kamut tortillas, crab meat, light cream cheese, cumin powder, curry powder, dried oregano, dried thyme leaves, dried mustard, eggs, extra virgin olive oil, feta cheese, white wine, parsley, garlic, garlic powder, granulated sugar, green chilies, ground black pepper, ground cinnamon, ground cloves, ground coriander, ground cumin, ground nutmeg, ground turkey, turkey breast, ground beef, lean chicken, honey, chili sauce, iceberg lettuce, cottage cheese, cabbage, valerian salad, red beans, pepper, low-fat milk, maple syrup, marjoram leaves, light mayonnaise, cottage cheese, mushrooms, sugar-free liquid cream, cannellini beans, nutmeg, onion powder, onions, parsley, pearl barley, quinoa, pineapple, pumpkin puree, oatmeal, mixed dry spices, oriental spices (Ras el Hanout), raspberries, red bell bell pepper, red chili powder, red onion, , rice flour, rice milk, sweet corn, onion, tomato sauce, pasture butter, unsalted tuna, vanilla extract, flour, whey protein powder, whipped topping, white onion, wild rice, Worcestershire sauce, zucchini.

Meal Plan Week 2

Day	Breakfast	Lunch	Dinner	Snacks/Sides	Smoothies
8	French Toast with Honey and Cinnamon	Beef and turkey sausages with lemon sauce	Barley and Beef Stew	Roasted Onion Dip	Blueberries and Coconut Smoothie
9	Breakfast Tacos	Celery Tuna Salad	Chicken and Corn Soup	Roasted Garlic White Bean Dip	Apple-Cinnamon Drink
10	Mexican Scrambled Eggs in Tortilla	Meat Casserole	Spicy vegetable stew	Green Goddess Dip	Blackberry-Sage Drink
11	American Blueberry Pancakes	Ground Beef in A Cup	Asparagus, Chicken and Wild Rice Soup	Crab and Carrot Dip	Apple Beet Juice Blend
12	Berries salad with Italian ricotta cheese	Spiced turkey breast with vegetables	Pumpkin Chili	Baba Ghanoush	Caramel Protein Latte
13	Summer Veggie Omelet	Quinoa Salad with Chickpeas and Feta	Cauliflower Manchurian	Spicy Kale Chips	Cinnamon Smoothie
14	Raspberry Overnight Porridge	Konjac spaghetti with broccoli and pine nuts	Green Asparagus Soup	Cinnamon Tortilla Chips	Raspberry and Pineapple Smoothie

Shopping List Week 3

Rye flour, almond butter, almond extract, almond milk, anchovies in oil, asparagus, baking powder, baking soda substitute, balsamic vinegar, banana, basil leaves, bean sprouts, blackberries, blueberries, Boston lettuce leaves, coffee, broccoli, brown sugar, brussels sprouts, buckwheat, butter, ghee, carrot, cayenne pepper, cherry tomatoes, chervil, chia seeds, chicken breast, chili pepper, chili powder, Chinese five-spice powder, coconut milk, ghee, corn tortillas, curry powder, spice blend, dill, dried sage, eggplant, egg, cucumber, extra virgin olive oil, flour tortillas, fresh basil, fresh bay leaf, fresh cilantro, fresh tarragon, fresh thyme, garlic, mustard, brown sugar, erythritol, grapefruit, Greek yogurt, green beans, green bell pepper, ground black pepper, ground coriander, ground cumin, honey, jalapeno bell pepper, cabbage, lemon, lemon pepper dressing, lettuce leaves, lime, lime leaf, low-fat milk, macadamia nuts, mango, maple extract, MCT oil, eggs, mint leaves, sugar free meringues, sugar free liquid cream, nutmeg, olive oil, onion, onion powder, oregano leaves, parmesan cheese, pears, pecans, pecorino romano, veal kidney, pine nuts, pineapple, plain cream cheese, popcorn, pure vanilla extract, canola oil, red apple, red peppers, red cabbage, red pepper, red onion, rice milk, pilaf rice, rosemary leaves, saffron, sage leaves salt, shallots, soy sauce, spinach, spring onions, stevia, strawberries, summer squash, sweet onion, tarragon, Thai red curry paste, thyme leaves, tomatoes, turkey breast, fat- fed unsalted butter, rice milk, vanilla whey protein powder, vegetable broth, vinegar, watercress, red potatoes, whey protein powder, whipped cream, whole wheat bread, white onion, white rice, white wine, yellow bell bell pepper, organic cornmeal, yellow squash, zucchini.

Meal Plan Week 3

Day	Breakfast	Lunch	Dinner	Snacks/Sides	Smoothies
15	Cheesy Scrambled Eggs with Fresh Herbs	Green Bean and Potato Salad	Pineapple and Pepper Curry	Sweet and Spicy Kettle Corn	Power-Boosting Smoothie
16	Turkey and spinach omelette	Chicken and Asparagus Salad with Watercress	Ratatouille	Meringue Cookies	Digestive Smoothie
17	Mexican Style Burritos	Chicken and Zucchini Salad with Nuts	Brussels Sprouts with Pears	Corn Bread	Strengthening Smoothie Bowl
18	Rye Flour Pancakes	Veal Kidneys	Stuffed Zucchini	Cucumber-Wrapped Vegetable Rolls	Antioxidant Berry Smoothie
19	Buckwheat and Grapefruit Porridge	Konjac spaghetti with broccoli and pine nuts	Thai Red Curry Vegetables and Rice	Chicken, pumpkin and onion skewers	Berry and Almond Smoothie
20	Egg and Veggie Muffins	Zucchini Risotto with Kidneys	Vegetable Paella	Chicken Lettuce Wraps	Mango and Pear Smoothie
21	Festive Berry Parfait	Spaghetti with zucchini and champignons	Eggplant Casserole	Antojitos	Keto Coffee Smoothie

Shopping List Week 4

Allspice, almond butter, almond milk, almonds, coconut milk, apple, apple cider vinegar, asparagus, coconut flour, almond flour, flaxseed, basil leaves, bay leaves, bread crumbs, brown sugar, pasture butter, canned chickpeas, carrots, celery, cherries, chia seeds, chicken broth, chicken thighs, chili, cinnamon, coconut cream, coconut flakes, coconut kefir, cornstarch, zucchini, blackberries, strawberries, raspberries, blueberries, cranberry juice, cream cheese, natural peanut butter, crystallized ginger, desalted capers, dried oregano, dried thyme, chicken wings, eggs, eggplant, extra virgin olive oil, flounder fillets, swordfish, canned tuna fillets, tortillas, fresh cilantro, fresh green beans, fresh chili, fresh oregano, fresh parsley, fresh rosemary, fresh thyme, garlic, garlic powder, ginger, brown sugar, erythritol, stevia, green olives, green onion, pear, rhubarb, ground black pepper, ground cumin, ground flaxseed, ground nutmeg, guanciale, hemp seeds, honey, chili sauce, jalapeno bell pepper,, cabbage, lean ground beef, lemon, light cheese, light sour cream, lime, basmati or long-grain rice, low-fat Greek yogurt, skim milk, mint leaves, mozzarella, fat-free lemon yogurt, onion, orange, green and red bell bell pepper, papaya, parmesan cheese, pecans, pecorino romano, pine nuts, pistachios, plain cream cheese, plums, pork leg, Konjac noodles, Konjac noodles, red or green grapes, low-fat pork sausage, low-sodium soy sauce, ripe peach, sage leaves, salt, shallots, stevia, sunflower seeds, sweet onion, sweet paprika, tomato sauce, tomatoes, celery, turnip, beet, carrot, sweet potato, unsweetened rice milk, vanilla, vanilla bean, vanilla bone broth protein powder, vanilla extract, wheat berries, hamburger buns, whole wheat, couscous, whole grain bread, zucchinis.

Meal Plan Week 4

Day	Breakfast	Lunch	Dinner	Snacks/Sides	Smoothies
22	Simple Chia Porridge	Asparagus in Salad with Poached Eggs	Ground Beef and Rice Soup	Roasted Onion Garlic Dip	Blackberry and Apple Smoothie
23	Rhubarb Bread Pudding	Swordfish steak with lime and celery salad	Couscous Burgers	Cheese-Herb Dip	Minty Cherry Smoothie
24	Fruit and Cheese Breakfast Wrap	Konjac spaghetti with broccoli	Baked Flounder	Zesty Chicken Wings	Vitaminic Coconut smoothie
25	Grandma Pancake Special	Rice & Tuna Salad with Mediterranean Pesto	Persian Chicken	Yogurt Fruit Dip	Green Minty Smoothie
26	Baked Frittata with lean meat	Gluten-free Pizza Margherita	Souvlaki Pork Skewers	Veggie Healthy Chips	Winter Berry Smoothie
27	Wheat Berry Breakfast Bowl	Spaghetti "Alla Norma"	Herbed Veal Meatloaf	Roasted Grapes	Carrot Smoothie
28	Breakfast Toast	Penne with and Basil	Chicken Stew	Spicy Strawberry Plums Peach Salsa	Strawberry Papaya Smoothie

Conclusion

Although the DASH diet was not at the time explicitly designed to lose weight, it is also suitable for this purpose.

And you should know that losing even a tiny bit of excess weight offers real health benefits. The DASH diet is rich in low-calorie foods such as fruits and vegetables, with various lean protein foods, and some with a healthy fatty acid content. You can further reduce the number and quality of calories consumed by replacing high-calorie foods like sweets with more fruits and vegetables, which makes it easier to achieve the goals of the DASH diet.

Did you not succeed?

Don't get down... and most of all, don't give up!

The DASH diet is a new way of eating and a diet that should be followed for life. If you don't follow it for a few days, don't be discouraged and continue to pursue your dietary goals and get back on the "straight and narrow". How? Let's find out together.

1. **Ask yourself why you were tempted**. Was there a party? Were you stressed about work or family life? Find out what caused your temporary deviation and get back on the DASH diet immediately.

2. **Don't worry too much**. Everyone on a diet will be tempted at some point, especially when they are still in the process of breaking in. Remember that changing your lifestyle is a process that can take a long time.

3. **Ask yourself whether you have tried to do too much at once**. Often people who try to change their lifestyle try to do too much: try to change a few things at a time. The change will be slower, but it is definitely the best way to succeed.

4. **Break the process into many small steps.** By doing this, not only will you not be tempted to do too much at once, but you will see that the changes are easier. Break one difficult task into many smaller and simpler steps, which are therefore much easier to accomplish.

5.   **Keep a diary**. Use a diary to keep a record of what you eat and what you do, which will make it much easier to see where the problem lies. Keep a diary for several days. You may find, for example, that you are in the habit of eating fatty foods while watching television, in which case you could start by keeping a less fatty snack substitute on hand. The diary will also help you determine whether you are eating a balanced diet and getting enough physical activity.

6.   **Celebrate success**. Give yourself a reward (that is not edible) every time you achieve a goal.

Start the DASH diet now: it can help prevent or control high blood pressure, but not only that, as it can benefit the heart, can be used as a weight-loss diet, and is well suited to any nutritional need.

I hope I have answered all your questions and thoughts running through your mind and that you are now enlightened...on your way to DASH! You'll see, it won't be difficult. You just need to put in these ingredients: your motivation and focus, a pinch of discipline, a bit of work and, of course, with this Dash diet cookbook as your guide, you will surely reach your goal!

Love,

yours Tara Cohen.